WORKBOOK TO ACCOMPANY
RESPIRATORY CARE ANATOMY AND PHYSIOLOGY
FOUNDATIONS FOR CLINICAL PRACTICE

Glenn Thom, BS, RRT

Assistant Director, Respiratory Care
St. Alexius Medical Center
Bismarck, North Dakota

Will Beachey, MEd, RRT

Assistant Professor and Program Director
School of Respiratory Care
St. Alexius Medical Center and the University of Mary
Bismarck, North Dakota

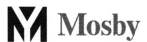

St. Louis   Baltimore   Boston   Carlsbad   Chicago   Minneapolis   New York   Philadelphia   Portland
London   Milan   Sydney   Tokyo   Toronto

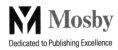
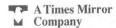

Vice President and Publisher: Don Ladig
Editor: Jennifer Roche
Managing Editor: Janet Russell
Project Manager: Gayle May Morris
Manufacturing Manager: Don Carlisle

Copyright © 1998 by Mosby–Year Book, Inc.

All rights reserved. No part of this publication may be reproduced, stored in a retrieval system, or transmitted, in any form or by any means, electronic, mechanical, photocopying, recording, or otherwise, without written permission of the publisher.

Permission to photocopy or reproduce solely for internal or personal use is permitted for libraries or other users registered with the Copyright Clearance Center, provided that the base fee of $4.00 per chapter plus $.10 per page is paid directly to the Copyright Clearance Center, 27 Congress Street, Salem, MA 01970. This consent does not extend to other kinds of copying, such as copying for general distribution, for advertising or promotional purposes, for creating new collected works, or for resale.

Printed in the United States of America
Composition by Black Dot Group
Printing/binding by Plus Communications

Mosby–Year Book, Inc.
11830 Westline Industrial Drive
St. Louis, Missouri 63146

International Standard Book Number: 0-8151-2582-8

97 98 99 00 01/9 8 7 6 5 4 3 2 1

Dedication
To Deb, Jess, and Mehl
Thanks for your patience and understanding!

Introduction

Respiratory care practitioners bring a variety of skills to the bedside. Critical thinking, the capstone of expertise in clinical skill, requires the bedside practitioner to identify, organize, and act on myriad pieces of clinical data. Each piece of clinical data represents a portion of the patient's physiologic status at a certain point in time. A strong knowledge base in respiratory care anatomy and physiology empowers the practitioner to validate diagnostic and therapeutic approaches to disease management, as indicated by clinical information.

As an adjunct to the text, *Respiratory Care Anatomy and Physiology*, this workbook allows the respiratory care student to reinforce essential core knowledge. Each chapter review is divided into four sections. "Points to Remember" highlights the most important "take home" learning objectives in the chapter. "The Basics" section includes matching, multiple choice, and fill-in-the-blank questions that provide a foundational review of the facts. The questions found in the "Putting It All Together" section assume that the student understands and is able to organize information presented in the current and previous chapters when responding to thought-provoking problems. The "Cases to Consider" section gives the student opportunities to apply their knowledge and critical thinking skills in a variety of clinical settings.

After completing these exercises, the student will have a working knowledge of respiratory care anatomy and physiology in health and disease. As each student builds on this knowledge base, they become practitioners who make significant contributions to positive patient outcomes.

Contents

Section I The Respiratory System

1. The Airways and Alveoli, *1*
2. The Lungs and Chest Wall, *9*
3. The Mechanics of Ventilation, *17*
4. Ventilation, *29*
5. Pulmonary Function Measurements, *35*
6. Pulmonary Blood Flow, *43*
7. Gas Diffusion, *51*
8. Oxygen Equilibrium and Transport, *58*
9. Carbon Dioxide Equilibrium and Transport, *65*
10. Acid-Base Regulation, *70*
11. Control of Ventilation, *76*
12. Ventilation-Perfusion Relationships and Arterial Blood Gases, *83*
13. Clinical Assessment of Acid-Base and Oxygenation Status, *90*

Section II The Cardiovascular System

14. Functional Anatomy of the Cardiovascular System, *106*
15. Cardiac Electrophysiology, *114*
16. The Electrocardiogram and Cardiac Arrhythmias, *122*
17. Control of Cardiac Output and Hemodynamics, *130*

Section III Integrated Function in Exercise

18. Cardiopulmonary Response to Exercise in Health, Disease, and Aging, *137*

Section IV The Renal System

19. Renal Regulation of Fluids, Electrolytes, and Acid-Base Balance, *144*

Answer Key, *152*

Chapter 1

Section I
The Respiratory System

The Airways and Alveoli

▷ Points to Remember

- Upper airway anatomy includes the nose, oral cavity, pharynx, and larynx. These components serve to humidify, warm, filter, and conduct inspired air to the lower airways.
- Lower airways are normally protected from aspiration by the function of the larynx and epiglottis.
- Vocal cords, while providing phonation for speech, are also a necessary part of the cough mechanism, essential in normal airway clearance.
- The trachea, mainstem bronchi, carina, and lobar, segmental, and subsegmental bronchi comprise the conducting airways. These airways remain patent (open) because of the presence of cartilaginous rings in their structure.
- The presence of bronchioles in the lung parenchyma (tissue), while part of the conducting airways, signals the beginning of non-cartilaginous airways.
- Terminal bronchioles, alveolar ducts, and alveoli comprise the acinus, the primary functional respiratory unit of the lung.
- The alveolar-capillary membrane is the structure across which gases from inspired air exchange with gases in the circulating blood.
- Smaller, gas-exchanging airways are kept patent by the parenchyma's elasticity and by the presence of alveolar surfactant.
- Important aspects of bronchial hygiene include properly conditioned inspired air, mucociliary clearance, large and small airway patency, and the cough mechanism.
- Aspirated material is more likely to enter the right lung than the left lung because the left mainstem bronchus angles more sharply away from the trachea's midline.
- Small airways less than two millimeters in diameter offer less resistance to airflow than larger upper airways because the collective cross-sectional area of small airways is greater.
- Mucus plugging of airways leads to atelectasis and hypoxemia.
- Water movement into the airways is an osmotic process controlled by epithelial chloride ion secretion, a mechanism that is defective in cystic fibrosis.
- The alveoli and lung interstitium depend on alveolar macrophage activity for lung clearance; poor macrophage clearance may lead to pulmonary interstitial fibrosis.

▶ The Basics

I. The Upper Airway

1. Label the following structures of the upper airway: middle meatus, superior meatus, inferior meatus, opening of auditory tube, hard palate, nasopharynx, soft palate, lingual tonsil, palantine tonsil, esophagus, trachea, cricoid cartilage, laryngopharynx, oropharynx, thyroid cartilage, vocal cord, and epiglottis.

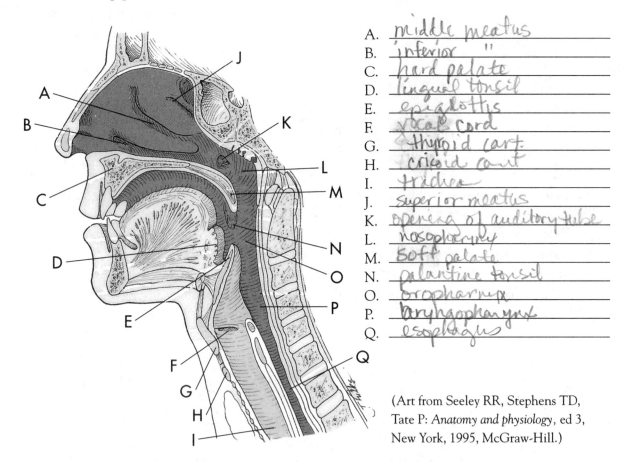

A. middle meatus
B. inferior "
C. hard palate
D. lingual tonsil
E. epiglottis
F. vocal cord
G. thyroid cart.
H. cricoid cart
I. trachea
J. superior meatus
K. opening of auditory tube
L. nasopharynx
M. soft palate
N. palantine tonsil
O. oropharynx
P. laryngopharynx
Q. esophagus

(Art from Seeley RR, Stephens TD, Tate P: *Anatomy and physiology*, ed 3, New York, 1995, McGraw-Hill.)

2. The nose alters inspired air by:
   A. Humidifing, cooling, and reducing flow velocity
   B. Cooling, filtering, and humidifying
   C. Humidifying, filtering, and warming
   D. Warming, reducing flow velocity, and filtering

3. The pharynx is composed of three subcomponents, named: naso-, oro-, and laryngo-.

4. Inspired infectious agents first encounter the immunologic defense of lymphatic tissue in the nasopharynx and oropharynx.

5. The most common threat to maintaining an open upper airway involves inappropriate positioning of the:
   A. Tongue
   B. Epiglottis
   C. Soft palate
   D. Tonsils

6. Label the structures associated with the vocal cords: thyroid cartilage, epiglottis, tracheal cartilage, false vocal cord, true vocal cords, arytenoid cartilage, corniculate cartilage, cricoid cartilage, glottis (or trachea), vallecula, cuneiform cartilage, and cricothyroid ligament.

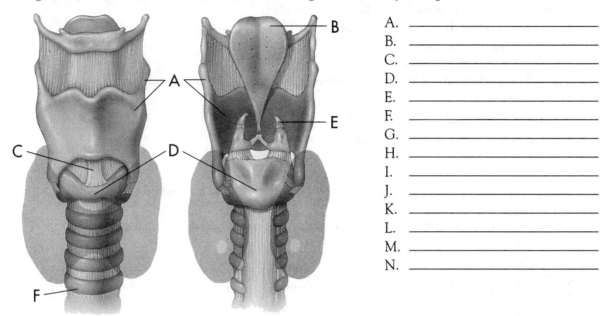

A. _____
B. _____
C. _____
D. _____
E. _____
F. _____
G. _____
H. _____
I. _____
J. _____
K. _____
L. _____
M. _____
N. _____

(Art from Seeley RR, Stephens TD, Tate P: *Anatomy and physiology*, ed 3, New York, 1995, McGraw-Hill.)

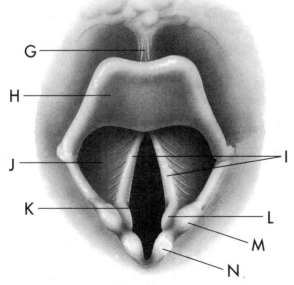

Chapter 1: The Airways and Alveoli   3

7. The _____ is called the "voice box" because it contains the vocal cords.

8. "Adam's apple" is the name sometimes given to the:
   A. Cricoid cartilage
   B. Thyroid cartilage
   C. Epiglottis
   D. Larynx

9. Vallecula is the name given to:
   A. The opening to the trachea
   B. An important landmark for tracheal tube insertion
   C. A flat leaf-shaped cartilage above the glottis
   D. A surgical opening into the trachea

10. The only complete ring of cartilage encircling the airway in the larynx or trachea is the:
    A. Cricoid cartilage
    B. Thyroid cartilage
    C. Epiglottis
    D. Larynx

11. The _____ form a triangular opening leading into the trachea.

12. Of the following, the structure essential in generating high pressure during a cough is the:
    A. Vallecula
    B. Epiglottis
    C. Cricothyroid ligament
    D. Vocal cords

13. In the larynx, _____ occurs if anything but air attempts to enter the airway.

II. The Lower Airways

Referring to the diagram and the text, answer questions 14 through 19.

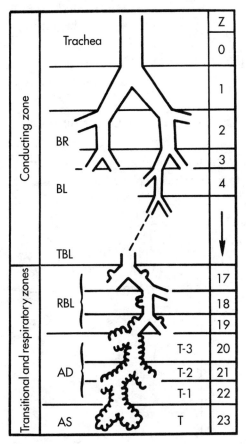

(Art modified from Weibel, ER: *Morphometry of the human lung*, Berlin, 1963, Springer-Verlag.)

14. Gas exchange between inspired air and circulating blood occurs in which zone?
    _____

15. Alveoli are located at level(s) _____.

16. Cartilage resembling that found at the trachea is also located in level(s)
    _____.

17. The ____Carina____ is the point of division for the mainstem bronchi. The external landmark for this division point is the ____5th____ thoracic vertebra.

18. The ____L____ mainstem bronchus divides more sharply from the trachea than the ____R____ mainstem bronchus.

19. Match the following lower airway structures with the appropriate statement:

   _____ Conducting airways   A. Elastic fibers forming lung tissue
   _____ Alveoli   B. Source of secretions in terminal bronchioles
   _____ Clara cells   C. Gas-exchanging sacs
   _____ Acinus   D. Mark the beginning of the gas exchange zone
   _____ Pores of Kohn   E. Airways that do not participate in gas exchange
   _____ Respiratory bronchioles   F. Connect adjacent alveoli
   _____ Parenchyma   G. Functional respiratory unit

III. The Cellular (Histologic) Composition of the Lower Airways

20. Label the cellular features of the following cross-sectional diagram: mucous blanket, goblet cell, adventitia, mucous gland, lamina propria, epithelium, mucosa, and submucosa.

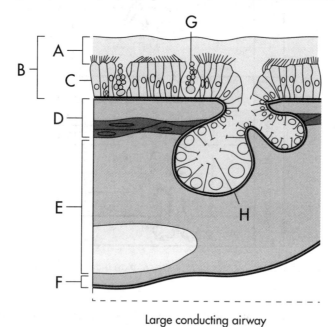

Large conducting airway

A. _____   E. _____
B. _____   F. _____
C. _____   G. _____
D. _____   H. _____

21. The mucous blanket is formed by secretions from the _____ cells and the _____ glands.

22. Epithelial cells called _____ move the sheet of mucus toward the pharynx.

23. The mucous blanket is composed of two layers. The upper component, which traps particles, is called the ____gel____ layer. The lower component, through which cilia move on the return stroke, is called the ____sol____ layer.

24. Mucus movement in the airway is known as:
    A. Viscoelasticity
    B. Atelectasis
    C. Ciliary dyskinesia
    D. Mucokinesis

25. Normal daily mucus production is about:
    A. 10 ml
    B. 50 ml
    C. 70 ml
    D. 100 ml

IV. The Gas Exchange Zone of the Lower Airways

26. Descending from the larger airways, alveoli first appear in the:
    A. Respiratory bronchioles
    B. Terminal bronchioles
    C. Conducting airways
    D. Bronchi

27. Most of the alveolar surface is comprised of:
    A. Serous cells
    B. Clara cells
    C. Type I cells
    D. Type II cells

▶ Putting It All Together

1. Patients requiring long-term ventilation often undergo a procedure called tracheotomy, during which a semi-permanent surgical opening (tracheostomy) is formed directly into the trachea. A short, curved tracheostomy tube is placed into this opening, through which the patient then breathes. You would expect that a patient with a recent tracheostomy would benefit most from:
   A. High airflows provided to the tracheal opening
   B. Dehumidified air provided to the airway
   C. A cool mist for adequate hydration
   D. Heated, humidified inspired air

2. Asthmatic patients frequently experience aggravated respiratory symptoms and also suffer from "head colds" or sinus infections. A logical explanation for this phenomenon is:
   A. Asthmatics are always prone to more viral infections.
   B. The trigger for sinusitis and asthma symptoms are always the same.
   C. Sinus drainage may be infecting the lungs and causing bronchospasm.
   D. Asthma attacks cause head colds.

3. Cardiopulmonary resuscitation is often done outside the hospital setting. An important technique in ventilating the patient involves tilting the victim's head back and thrusting the jaw forward. This is done to allow:
   A. Better blood flow to the head
   B. Air forced into the mouth easier passage to the lungs
   C. Easier mouth alignment
   D. Reducing the chance of damage to the upper airways

4. Cromolyn sodium is a drug inhaled into the airways to inhibit mast cell breakdown. This drug would be most useful in treating:
   A. Cystic fibrosis
   B. Ciliary dyskinesia
   C. Allergic asthma
   D. Emphysema

5. Certain lung diseases impair the alveolar-capillary membrane's gas-diffusing capabilities. An important consequence of this would be:
   A. A decrease in blood oxygen levels
   B. A decrease in blood carbon dioxide levels
   C. An increase in blood oxygen levels
   D. An increase in blood oxygen and carbon dioxide levels

6. In the adult respiratory distress syndrome (ARDS), the permeability of the alveolar-capillary membrane is increased. These patients would probably have:
   A. Higher than normal oxygen blood levels
   B. Hyperinflated alveoli
   C. Impermeability of "tight junctions" increased
   D. Increased fluid in the alveoli

7. Because of damage to the lung parenchyma in ARDS, levels of surfactant in the alveoli are reduced. It is not unusual for ARDS patients to require mechanical ventilation. One would expect the ventilator pressure required to deliver each breath to be:
   A. Higher than normally required
   B. Less than normally required
   C. Equal to that normally required
   D. Unaffected by the presence of ARDS

▶ A Case to Consider

You are a respiratory therapist completing your final check for the evening. As you enter the next patient room, your patient appears to be sleeping soundly. Since this patient is receiving oxygen, you want to approach the bed and ensure the proper liter flow on the wall flowmeter before leaving quietly. When at the bedside, you notice the patient's abdomen is making ventilatory movements, but no breathing is audible. On closer inspection, you feel no air movement from the nose or mouth. What are your initial suspicions?

Chapter 2

The Lungs and Chest Wall

▶ Points to Remember

- The heart, aorta, esophagus, great veins, trachea, and mainstem bronchi are contained between the lungs in the mediastinum.
- The diaphragm is the major muscle of ventilation.
- Arteries, veins, and bronchi enter and leave the lungs at a point called the hilum.
- The membrane in contact with the lung is the visceral pleura; it is continuous with the membrane attached to the chest wall, the parietal pleura.
- Fluid in the potential space between the visceral and parietal pleura allows for free movement between the lung surface and the chest wall.
- Pulmonary arteries carry oxygen-poor blood from the heart, and pulmonary veins carry oxygenated blood back to the heart.
- The vertebrae, sternum, diaphragm, and ribs form the thoracic cavity.
- The twelve ribs include seven vertebrosternal, three vertebrochondral, and two floating ribs.
- The sternum has three parts: the manubrium, body, and xiphoid process. The sternal angle (angle of Louis) marks the position of the carina.
- Ventilation is facilitated, in part, by "bucket handle" and "pump handle" movements of the ribs at their attachments to the sternum and spinal column.
- Intercostal and scalene muscles assist the diaphragm in quiet breathing.
- Accessory muscles (sternomastoids, pectoralis major, and abdominals) are used in periods of increased ventilatory demand.
- Somatic nerves provide for ventilatory innervation. Damage to the spine in this area often results in ventilatory impairment.
- All sensory and motor innervation to the lung is autonomic (involuntary) and is supplied by the vagus nerve.
- The autonomic system is divided into the sympathetic, parasympathetic, nonadrenergic-noncholinergic stimulatory, and nonadrenergic-noncholinergic inhibitory systems.
- Airways are innervated by parasympathetic fibers but not sympathetic fibers; however, airways do contain sympathetic receptors.
- Stimulation of airway adrenergic receptors by circulating norepinephrine causes smooth muscle relaxation and bronchodilation and secretion thinning.

- Stimulation of cholinergic fibers causes smooth muscle contraction and bronchospasm; the viscosity of secretions is also increased.
- Nitric oxide is the neurotransmitter for the non-adrenergic non-cholinergic nervous system.
- The cough reflex, an essential part of bronchial hygiene, is a sequential action involving diaphragmatic contraction, inspiratory pause, glottis closure, abdominal muscle contraction, and glottis opening.

▶ The Basics

I. Anatomy

1. Label the organs and landmarks associated with the lungs: thyroid cartilage, liver, sternum, trachea, right heart border, stomach, lung apex, right diaphragm border, cardiac notch, left heart border, left diaphragm border, and clavicle.

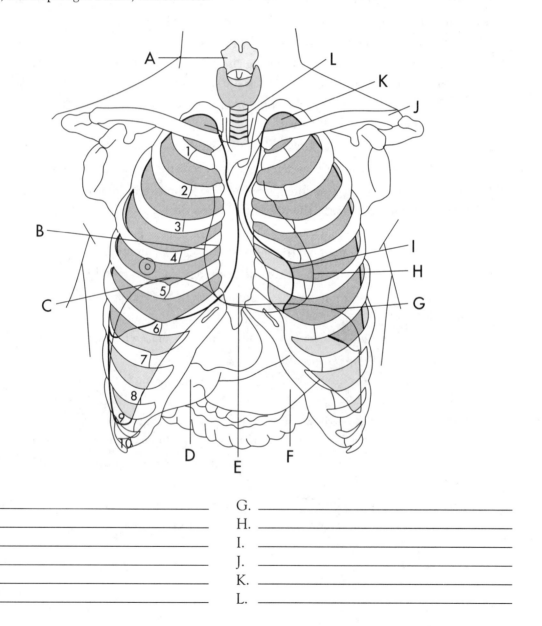

A. _____
B. _____
C. _____
D. _____
E. _____
F. _____
G. _____
H. _____
I. _____
J. _____
K. _____
L. _____

2. The heart, aorta, esophagus, great veins, trachea, and mainstem bronchi are contained in the:
   A. Pleural space
   B. Mediastinum
   C. Apex
   D. Cardiac notch

3. The major muscle(s) of ventilation is (are) called the:
   A. Pulmonary ligament
   B. Scalenes
   C. Abdominals
   D. Diaphragm

4. The left diaphragmatic surface is lower than the right because the _____ rests on the left and the _____ props up the right.

5. Label the parts of the thoracic cavity: parietal pleura, diaphragm, thyroid cartilage, right bronchus, left bronchus, visceral pleura, trachea, larynx, cricoid cartilage, aorta, mediastinum, and pleural space.

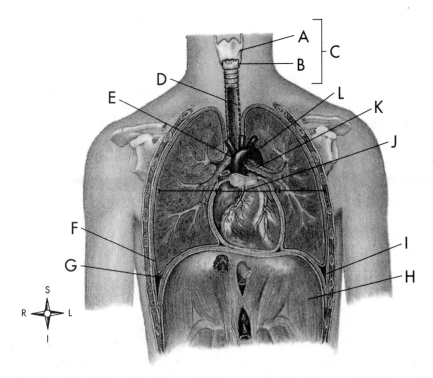

(Art from Thibodeau GA, Patton KT: *Anatomy and physiology*, ed 3, St Louis, Mosby.)

A. _____
B. _____
C. _____
D. _____
E. _____
F. _____
G. _____
H. _____
I. _____
J. _____
K. _____
L. _____

6. Match the phrases on the left with the most appropriate terminology on the right:
   _____ Connects visceral pleura with diaphragm
   _____ Left lung portion overlapping heart
   _____ Attached to inner chest wall surface
   _____ Between visceral and parietal membranes
   _____ Diaphragm meets chest wall
   _____ Result of inflamed pleural space
   _____ Tube in pleural cavity
   _____ Air in pleural space

   A. Pleural space
   B. Costophrenic angle
   C. Thoracentesis
   D. Pulmonary ligament
   E. Pneumothorax
   F. Pleural effusion
   G. Lingula
   H. Parietal pleura

7. The origin of the pulmonary circulation is the:
   A. Pulmonary artery
   B. Pulmonary vein
   C. Bronchial artery
   D. Bronchopulmonary anastomosis

8. Airway walls in the lung receive blood from the:
   A. Pulmonary arteries
   B. Pulmonary veins
   C. Bronchial arteries
   D. Bronchopulmonary anastomoses

II. Circulation

9. Mixing of oxygenated and oxygen-poor blood occurs in the pulmonary circulatory system in the:
   A. Pulmonary arteries
   B. Pulmonary veins
   C. Bronchial arteries
   D. Bronchopulmonary anastomoses

10. Oxygen-poor blood is carried from the heart to the lungs by the:
    A. Pulmonary artery
    B. Pulmonary vein
    C. Bronchial artery
    D. Bronchopulmonary anastomosis

11. Shunting (mixing of oxygen-poor blood with oxygenated blood) in pulmonary veins means the partial pressure (concentration) of oxygen in alveolar air will always be (higher, lower) than in blood leaving the lung.

12. Fluid removal and filtering in interstitial spaces (spaces between cells and vessels) is accomplished in the lungs by the:
    A. Pulmonary circulation
    B. Lymphatic system
    C. True bronchial veins
    D. Pleural space

III. Innervation

13. Indicate whether each of the following is representative of the somatic ("S") or autonomic ("A") nervous system:

    _____ Chest wall muscles _____ Phrenic nerves
    _____ Lung _____ Diaphragm
    _____ Airway smooth muscle _____ Vagus nerve
    _____ Voluntary motor control _____ Intercostal nerves

14. Current theory about the autonomic innervation of airways involves four separate components: the _____ system; the _____ system; the _____ inhibitory system; and the _____ stimulatory fibers.

15. Stimulation of parasympathetic fibers produces all of the following *except*:
    A. Smooth muscle control
    B. Airway smooth muscle tone
    C. Mucous gland activity
    D. Thin secretions

16. Bronchospasm can be the result of:
    A. Overstimulation of smooth airway muscle nerve fibers
    B. Stimulation of adrenergic receptors
    C. Increased circulating epinephrine
    D. Stimulation of beta-2 receptors

17. The non-adrenergic, non-cholinergic (NANC) neurotransmitter is:
    A. Cyclic GMP
    B. Epinephrine
    C. Acetylcholine
    D. Nitric oxide

18. Nerve fibers leaving the spinal cord form synapses at nerve junctions. These junctions are called:
    A. Preganglionic fibers
    B. Ganglia
    C. Pulmonary plexus
    D. Postganglionic fibers

19. Match terms and descriptions of afferent nerves and responses:

    _____ Vagus
    _____ Deep inspiration
    _____ Slowly adapting receptors
    _____ Rapidly adapting receptors
    _____ Cough reflex
    _____ J-receptors
    _____ C-fiber receptors

    A. Located in epithelium of larynx, trachea, mainstem bronchi
    B. Origin of most afferent nerves
    C. Located in parenchyma, conducting airways, and pulmonary vasculature
    D. Located near capillaries and alveoli
    E. Part of Hering-Breuer reflex
    F. Stretch receptors in conducting airway smooth muscle
    G. Induced by stimulating large airway irritant receptors

IV. Muscles and Rib Cage

20. Number the proper sequence in the production of a cough:
    _____ Abdominal muscles contract forcefully
    _____ Diaphragm contracts
    _____ Glottis opens suddenly
    _____ Larynx muscles close the glottis
    _____ Inspiratory pause

21. Rib movement occurs in two ways, the _____ motion, in which sternal rib ends are elevated, and the _____ movement, in which the sternal and vertebral rib ends remain stationary.

22. The major muscle(s) active in quiet breathing is (are) the:
    A. Abdominals
    B. Pectoralis
    C. Diaphragm
    D. Intercostal

23. Accessory muscles of inspiration that elevate the sternum include the:
    A. Diaphragm and intercostals
    B. Intercostals
    C. Sternomastoid
    D. Intercostals and sternomastoid

24. The accessory muscles elevating and fixing the first and second ribs are called:
    A. Sternomastoid
    B. External intercostals
    C. Scalene
    D. Internal intercostals

25. The abdominal muscles are unique because they are the:
    A. Only accessory muscles of inspiration
    B. Only accessory muscles of expiration
    C. Accessory muscles active during quiet breathing
    D. Muscles assisting in inspiration at rest

26. Match each term with the most appropriate description about the ribs:
    _____ Floating   A. Immediately below the sternal angle
    _____ Vertebrosternal   B. Carina landmark
    _____ Vertebrochondral C. Ribs 11 and 12
    _____ Costal groove   D. Ribs 8, 9, and 10
    _____ Manubrium   E. Location of nerves, arteries, and veins
    _____ Body   F. Ribs 1 through 7
    _____ Xiphoid   G. Use caution during CPR
    _____ Angle of Louis   H. Immediately above sternal angle

▶ Putting It All Together

1. Inhaled ipratropium bromide inhibits parasympathetic stimulation. Patients with obstructive airways disease benefit from this drug because it:
   A. Increases secretion production
   B. Stimulates adrenergic receptors
   C. Decreases secretion viscosity
   D. Increases the quantity of mucoglycoproteins

2. Parasympathetic stimulation causes bronchoconstriction. Sympathetic stimulation causes bronchodilation. Parasympathetic inhibitors are used to relieve bronchoconstriction. Additional bronchodilatory effects could be expected when adding:
   A. A cholinergic stimulator
   B. A nitric oxide inhibitor
   C. A sympathetic inhibitor
   D. An adrenergic stimulator

3. Severe reactions to allergens (anaphylaxis) can often be relieved with self-administered epinephrine (from an "epi-pen"). Reversal of anaphylaxis occurs because epinephrine:
   A. Reverses parasympathetic stimulation
   B. Stimulates parasympathetic receptors
   C. Reverses sympathetic stimulation
   D. Stimulates adrenergic receptors

4. Inhaled methacholine is known to cause parasympathetic bronchoconstriction in asthmatic patients. Even though airway compromise from bronchoconstriction is undesirable, this chemical is used for testing pulmonary function. Why?
   A. It can help detect hyperreactive airways.
   B. It improves expiratory airflows.
   C. It reverses sympathetic stimulation.
   D. It assists in evaluating lung volumes.

5. A physiologic parameter known as "minute ventilation" is calculated by multiplying the volume of each breath (tidal volume) by the respiratory rate. It is possible for the minute ventilation of a patient developing a large pleural effusion to remain unchanged. Why?
   A. A higher respiratory rate can help offset the effects of reduced lung volume.
   B. Minute ventilation is unaffected by a pleural effusion.
   C. Lung volumes always remain constant.
   D. A pleural effusion will cause an increase in lung volumes, depressing the respiratory rate.

6. In addition to bronchospasm, nerves mediating increased airway smooth muscle tone also cause:
   A. Decreased work of breathing
   B. Difficulty in mucus clearance
   C. Improved mucus clearance
   D. Increased airflows

7. Comatose patients often lose irritant receptor response. As a result, these patients would probably be at increased risk for:
   A. Pleural effusions
   B. Bronchoconstriction
   C. Excessive coughing
   D. Aspiration of foreign material

8. An obese individual with a large abdomen may exhibit a shallow respiratory pattern (small tidal volumes) at rest. What would be the most likely reason?
   A. Asthma is probable with obesity.
   B. Diaphragmatic movement is limited.
   C. Increased physical exertion is present even at rest.
   D. Abnormal respiratory musculature is present.

9. A patient with advanced, severe chronic obstructive pulmonary disease (COPD) is leaning on a bedside table, grasping its edges while breathing at rest. Scalene and sternomastoid muscle activity is visible. These observations indicate:
   A. Probable nerve damage to the diaphragm
   B. A normal respiratory pattern
   C. Increased work of breathing
   D. Reduced work of breathing

▶ Cases to Consider

1. You have been asked to evaluate a patient who "doesn't like doctors" and has never had a comprehensive clinical evaluation. You make several observations as you enter the patient's room. The patient's shoulders seem to be fixed in an elevated state. Neck muscles are tensing with ventilation at rest. You read the radiologist's chest x-ray report before entering the room and noted the chest film exhibits a "flat" diaphragm and "hyperinflation." Based on these initial findings, you suspect the patient's clinical summary will probably include what diagnosis?

2. A respiratory care practitioner is treating a patient with very viscous pulmonary secretions. Inhaled acetylcysteine, a known airway irritant, is being used because of its secretion-thinning properties. During the treatment, the patient begins to wheeze noticeably and the wheezing does not diminish after secretions are expectorated. The practitioner realizes that a second inhaled drug must be added to the regimen. What type of drug should this be and what brought her to this conclusion?

Chapter 3

The Mechanics of Ventilation

▷ Points To Remember

- Resting lung volume (the functional residual capacity) is maintained by a balance between the outward recoil of the rib cage and the inward recoil of the lungs.
- Contact between the lungs and the rib cage is maintained by the negative pressure and film of fluid between the continuous visceral and parietal pleura.
- Compliance is a measure of opposition to lung inflation. It is measured as the change in lung volume per unit of pressure change (L/cm H_2O).
- Peak inspiratory pressure (PIP) is the pressure required to overcome airway resistance and elastic recoil. The difference between peak and plateau pressures is the pressure required to overcome airway resistance alone.
- Airway diameter is the most powerful factor influencing airway resistance.
- Airflow into and out of the lung occurs because pressure gradients are created by ventilatory musculature or positive-pressure mechanical ventilation.
- Large, branching airways typically exhibit turbulent airflow, while small, peripheral airways have laminar flow.
- Total lung capacity (TLC) is the amount of gas the lung contains at maximum inspiration.
- Basic, non-overlapping subdivisions of the TLC are known as *volumes*; the term *capacity* refers to the sum of two or more volumes.
- Regional differences in ventilation, volume, and compliance exist in the lung. Apical regions have a larger resting volume, lower compliance, and decreased ventilation as compared to basal regions.
- A time constant (TC) is an indicator of how long it takes to passively inflate or deflate the lung.
- Patients with long time constants tend to exhale incompletely, especially at fast breathing rates; this leads to air trapping and auto-PEEP.
- The equal pressure point (EPP) in the airways occurs when pressure outside the airway (pleural pressure) equals pressure inside the airway. Beyond EPP (toward the mouth) airways are compressed or collapsed.

- The appearance of the EPP at low lung volumes (less than 80% of vital capacity) limits maximal achievable expiratory flow rate; flow rates are effort independent under these circumstances.
- Patients with airflow obstruction tend to breathe slowly and deeply. Patients with low lung compliance tend to breathe rapidly and shallowly.
- Deformities of the thoracic cage can reduce total compliance and have a restrictive effect on ventilation parameters.
- Pulmonary surfactant reduces alveolar surface tension, preventing alveolar collapse and decreasing the work of breathing.
- Respiratory distress syndromes are disease states characterized by low surfactant levels and high elastic work of breathing.
- Signs of respiratory muscle fatigue and impending ventilatory failure include asynchrony (abdominal expansion lags behind chest expansion), paradoxical breathing (the abdomen moves inward on inspiration), and high frequency-to-tidal volume ratios (>100).

▶ The Basics

I. Static Lung-Chest Wall Mechanics

1. Match definitions with proper terms for lung-chest wall mechanics:

   _____ Recoil force
   _____ Contributes most to lung elasticity
   _____ Mouth pressure during spontaneous breathing
   _____ Alveolar pressure
   _____ Pressure between chest wall and lung
   _____ Difference between two pressures
   _____ No flow of air
   _____ Alveolar minus atmospheric pressure
   _____ Alveolar minus pleural pressure
   _____ Intrapleural minus atmospheric pressure

   A. Atmospheric pressure
   B. Intrapulmonary pressure
   C. Pressure gradient
   D. Elasticity
   E. Transpulmonary pressure
   F. Surface tension
   G. Transrespiratory pressure
   H. Transthoracic pressure
   I. Intrapleural pressure
   J. Zero pressure gradient

2. Label the ventilation pressures diagram on p. 19 appropriately: airway opening, body surface, transpulmonary, transrespiratory, intrapleural, alveolar, and transthoracic pressures.

A. _____ E. _____
B. _____ F. _____
C. _____ G. _____
D. _____

3. During expiration, alveolar pressure:
   A. Decreases, then increases
   B. Is above atmospheric pressure
   C. Is below atmospheric pressure
   D. Is equal to zero

4. Throughout the respiratory cycle, esophageal pressure is expected to:
   A. Remain elevated
   B. Closely follow pleural pressure
   C. Be unaffected
   D. Cancel out pleural pressure

5. As volume in the thorax begins to decrease during expiration, intrapleural pressure can be expected to:
   A. Increase
   B. Decrease
   C. Remain unchanged
   D. Decrease, then increase

6. Match the following terms with the appropriate descriptions:
   _____ Capacity
   _____ Volume
   _____ Total lung capacity
   _____ Residual volume
   _____ Vital capacity
   _____ Inspiratory capacity
   _____ Expiratory reserve volume
   _____ Functional residual capacity
   _____ Tidal volume

   A. Maximum limit of ventilation
   B. Comprised of at least two volumes
   C. Maximum inspiratory lung volume from end-tidal level
   D. Normal breath
   E. Exhalable volume beyond resting end-tidal level
   F. Cannot be exhaled
   G. Volume remaining in the lung at end-tidal exhalation
   H. Subdivision of a capacity
   I. Sum of all volumes

Chapter 3: The Mechanics of Ventilation   19

7. Maximum inspiratory pressure (MIP) and maximum expiratory pressure (MEP) are indicators of ventilatory muscle strength. The method for measuring these pressures primarily involves:
   A. Normal breathing effort
   B. Normal breathing through an open tube
   C. Maximum breathing effort through an occluded tube
   D. Maximum breathing effort through an open tube

8. Measurement of MIP and MEP should be done at specific lung volumes because of the state of the ventilatory musculature at these volumes. These volumes include:
   A. Residual volume and end-tidal volume
   B. Total lung capacity and functional residual capacity
   C. Residual volume and total lung capacity
   D. End-tidal volume and functional residual capacity

9. Ventilatory muscle strength is insufficient to sustain spontaneous ventilation when MIP generated is not stronger than an inspiratory pressure of:
   A. 50 cm H_2O
   B. -25 cm H_2O
   C. -75 cm H_2O
   D. 25 cm H_2O

Refer to the figure below for questions 10 through 13.

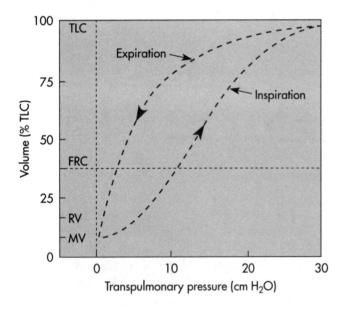

(Art from Berne RM, Levy MN: *Physiology*, ed 3, St Louis, 1993, Mosby.)

10. In the figure above, the inspiratory and expiratory limbs of the pressure-volume curve are different. This is known as hysteresis, which, in the lung, is due to:
    A. The elastic limit
    B. Hooke's law
    C. Alveolar surface tension
    D. Elastic tissue forces

11. Compare the pressure-volume relationship in the lower part of the pressure-volume loop (above FRC) to that in the upper part (close to TLC). The volume obtained per unit of pressure in the lower part of the loop is:
    A. Very close to that in the upper part
    B. The same as that in the upper part
    C. Less than that in the upper part
    D. Greater than that in the upper part

12. If the effects of alveolar surface tension and lung fiber characteristics were not present, the pressure-volume graph would:
    A. Be inverted
    B. Have greater distance between inspiratory and expiratory paths
    C. Have identical inspiratory and expiratory paths
    D. Have straight lines for inspiratory and expiratory paths

13. The pressure-volume curve is also known as a compliance curve. Compliance is defined as:
    A. Change in pressure per unit of volume
    B. Change in volume per unit of pressure
    C. Elastance
    D. Recoil force

Refer to the figure below to answer questions 14 and 15.

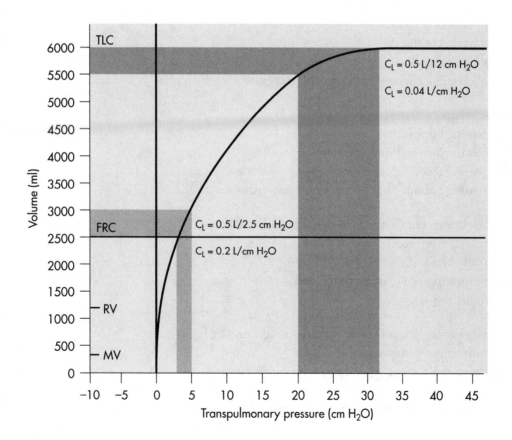

14. In the static compliance curve on p. 21, compliance at the end of a normal tidal volume is:
    A. Zero
    B. 0.04 L/cm H_2O
    C. Equal to compliance at residual volume
    D. Greater than compliance at total lung capacity

15. The static compliance curve indicates volume (increases, decreases) as pressure increases.

16. From total lung capacity (TLC), expired volume per unit of pressure will be less than inspired volume per unit of pressure near TLC because of alveolar surface tension. This phenomenon is called:
    A. Compliance
    B. Hooke's law
    C. Hysteresis
    D. Abnormal

17. Compliance is the opposite of:
    A. Distensibility
    B. Ease of inflation
    C. Elastance
    D. Volume changes with pressure changes

18. Emphysema is characterized by:
    A. High lung compliance
    B. Low lung compliance
    C. High lung recoil
    D. Small volume changes with pressure increases

19. Fibrosis affects the lung by:
    A. Increasing compliance
    B. Increasing distensibility
    C. Increasing recoil forces
    D. Increasing volume changes with pressure increases

20. Select the statement that *is not* associated with atelectasis.
    A. Increased lung recoil
    B. Low alveolar surface tension
    C. High intermolecular attraction forces
    D. Alveolar collapse

21. If critical opening pressure of an alveolus is abnormally high, then:
    A. The alveolus opens sooner
    B. The alveolus remains open longer during deflation
    C. The alveolar radius is increased
    D. The critical closing pressure is also increased

22. Surfactant is a natural substance present on the surface of alveolar fluid. A lung with abnormally low surfactant levels would be characterized by:
    A. Lower pressures to open alveoli
    B. Decreased surface tension
    C. Increased work of breathing
    D. Fewer atelectatic alveoli

II. Dynamic Lung-Chest Wall Mechanics

23. Match the following terms about dynamic lung-chest wall mechanics with the appropriate descriptions:

    _____ Driving pressure
    _____ Viscosity
    _____ Laminar flow
    _____ Turbulent flow
    _____ Poiseuille's law
    _____ Transitional flow

    A. Frictional resistance between gas molecules
    B. Pressure gradient
    C. High-velocity gas molecules impact airway walls frequently
    D. Pressure increases exponentially when airway radius decreases
    E. Flow occurring where airways branch
    F. Overlapping cylindrical gas layers moving at different speeds

24. Total compliance is decreased in kyphoscoliosis, a skeletal deformity. This is primarily due to:
    A. Decreased lung compliance
    B. A reduction in thoracic compliance
    C. Reduced recoil pressure
    D. A "stiffer" parenchyma

25. Resting volume of the lung-thorax system (functional residual capacity) is the product of:
    A. Thoracic recoil
    B. Lung recoil
    C. Unstressed thoracic resting volume
    D. Thoracic recoil and lung recoil

26. When the thorax component of the lung-thorax system is at rest, lung volume is:
    A. About 30% of vital capacity
    B. The same as unstressed resting lung volume
    C. About 70% of vital capacity
    D. Maximized

27. During a normal breath, airway resistance:
    A. Is less than at total lung capacity
    B. Increases during inspiration
    C. Decreases during inspiration
    D. Does not change

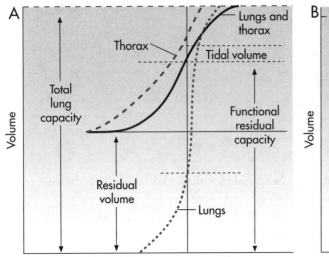
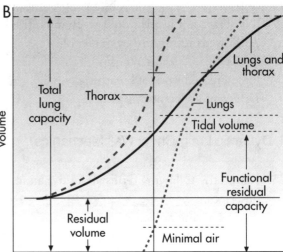
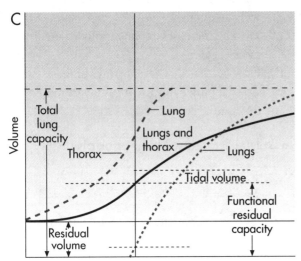

28. Refer to the diagrams above and indicate which diagram (A, B, or C) describes each statement best.

_____ Total compliance is decreased.
_____ Total compliance is increased.
_____ Residual volume percent of total lung capacity is increased.
_____ Lung compliance is normal.
_____ Lung compliance is increased.
_____ Lung compliance is consistent with chronic obstructive pulmonary disease.
_____ Lung compliance is consistent with fibrotic lung disease.
_____ High lung recoil force is present.
_____ Low lung recoil force is present.

29. Peak inspiratory pressure differs from plateau pressure in that it is:
    A. Generated by both airway resistance and lung elastic recoil
    B. Generated by lung elastic recoil
    C. Generated by airway resistance
    D. A measurement of compliance

30. In patients with abnormally high lung compliance, airway compression during an exhaled vital capacity:
    A. Does not occur
    B. Occurs later than in people with normal compliance
    C. Is unchanged from a normal lung
    D. Occurs earlier than in people with normal compliance

31. As pressure is applied to the trachea, the lungs expand until lung pressure equals applied pressure. The volume at this point will be determined primarily by:
    A. Inspiratory time
    B. Lung compliance
    C. Airway resistance
    D. All of the above

32. The time required to attain equalization of applied pressure and lung pressure is determined by:
    A. Airway resistance
    B. Lung compliance
    C. Both A and B
    D. Neither A nor B

33. Positive end-expiratory pressure (PEEP) occurs when lung units do not have adequate expiratory time to empty normally, causing them to maintain a positive pressure. PEEP changes lung volumes by:
    A. Decreasing the residual volume
    B. Increasing the functional residual capacity
    C. Decreasing the volume of tidal breathing
    D. Increasing compliance

34. In a normal lung, inspiration begins with alveolar pressure dropping slightly below mouth pressure, causing a pressure gradient and inspiratory airflow. How would the presence of auto-PEEP change normal inspiration?
    A. The mouth pressure-alveolar pressure gradient would be reduced.
    B. Inspiratory airflow would begin sooner in the cycle.
    C. Greater inspiratory effort would be required to generate a pressure gradient.
    D. Work of breathing would be reduced.

35. Regional differences in gas distribution in the lung are caused by the gravitational effects of lung tissue and blood on alveoli. These differences result in:
    A. Poorly ventilated apical regions
    B. Poor compliance in basal alveoli
    C. Less negative apical pleural pressure
    D. Lower apical alveolar recoil

▶ Putting It All Together

1. "Spontaneous" pneumothorax is a lung collapse occurring without any extrinsic trauma to the chest. Spontaneous pneumothoraces occur more often in the apices of the lungs than in other regions. Why would this be so?

2. Theophylline is a drug used in the management of chronic obstructive pulmonary disease because of its influence on the diaphragm. Which one of the following is a beneficial effect of theophylline on the diaphragm of the patient with COPD?
   A. The diaphragm is positioned lower at rest.
   B. Diaphragmatic oxygen consumption is increased.
   C. Diaphragmatic excursion is reduced.
   D. Diaphragmatic contractility is increased.

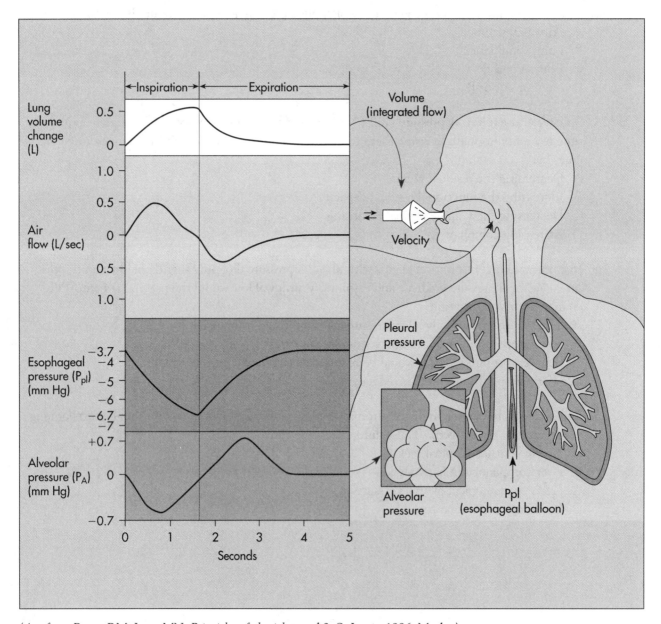

(Art from Berne RM, Levy MN: *Principles of physiology*, ed 2, St Louis, 1996, Mosby.)

26 The Respiratory System

Referring to the figure on p. 26, answer questions 3 through 5.

3. The spirogram and pressure measurements are for a patient with normal lungs. Select *all* of the following that represent expected abnormalities of a patient with fibrotic lung disease.
   A. Lung volume is increased.
   B. Lung volume is normal.
   C. Expiratory time is shortened.
   D. Expiratory airflow velocity is increased.
   E. Inspiratory pleural negative pressure is normal.
   F. Inspiratory pleural negative pressure is increased.
   G. End-expiratory alveolar pressure (no flow) is increased.
   H. End-expiratory alveolar pressure (no flow) is atmospheric.

4. Which variance from normal would you *not* expect in the lung dynamics of a patient with emphysema?
   A. Increased end-expiratory alveolar pressure
   B. Shortened expiratory time
   C. Reduced expiratory flow velocity
   D. Increased expiratory intrapleural pressure

5. Which would be true in a patient with diaphragmatic impairment?
   A. Inspiratory alveolar pressure would be less negative.
   B. Inspiratory airflow velocity would increase.
   C. Inspiratory lung volume would increase.
   D. Inspiratory esophageal pressure would be more negative.

6. Some mechanical ventilators are volume-limited. Breath-to-breath volumes delivered to the patient are essentially identical. If a patient's lung compliance decreased, the inspiratory positive pressure required to deliver a mechanical breath would be:
   A. Decreased
   B. Unchanged
   C. Increased
   D. Unrelated to compliance changes

7. An essential component of the cough effort is the ability to increase lung volume prior to forceful expulsion of inspired air. Patients with obstructive airways disease often have a large total lung capacity yet they experience difficulty expectorating secretions. The reasons for this include:
   A. Premature airway collapse during forceful expiration
   B. A reduction in functional residual capacity
   C. Increased lung elastic recoil
   D. A reduced equilibrium point for the functional residual capacity

8. According to Poiseuille's law, if a bronchogenic tumor compressed a mainstem bronchus to one-half its original diameter, the pressure required to maintain normal ventilation in the affected lung would:
   A. Be unchanged
   B. Double
   C. Be multiplied eight times
   D. Be multiplied sixteen times

9. Breath sounds such as wheezing indicate obstruction in the airways. These sounds are noisier than normal breath sounds because they are produced by:
   A. Lower velocity airflow
   B. Turbulent airflow
   C. Laminar airflow
   D. A low driving pressure

10. The respiratory care practitioner treating a mechanically ventilated patient with a large pleural effusion notices steadily increasing peak airway pressures. The practitioner asks the attending pulmonologist to consider a thoracentesis, which will remove most of the additional fluid in the pleural space. The practitioner believes that:
    A. Pleural fluid is reducing large airway diameter
    B. Removing the extra fluid will increase lung elasticity
    C. Pleural fluid is reducing lung distensibility
    D. Pleural fluid removal will lower airway resistance

▶ Cases to Consider

1. A respiratory care practitioner is managing a patient receiving mechanical ventilation. The patient has been suctioned for pulmonary secretions as needed, and breath sounds are clear with no evidence of secretions in the airways. A routine check of ventilator-patient parameters is being completed. As the practitioner notices that the peak inspiratory pressure and plateau pressure difference is significantly greater, the bedside nurse announces that the patient is having a seizure. The patient is experiencing visible, involuntary muscle contractions. The respiratory care practitioner realizes a "bite block" should be placed between the teeth of the patient to maintain adequate ventilation. Since an artificial airway is already in place, why is the bite block necessary?

2. Guillain-Barré is a disease characterized by progressive muscle weakness and paralysis. Respiratory care practitioners are concerned about a Guillain-Barré patient's ability to breathe and make certain measurements that help monitor ventilatory impairment. Why is ventilation a concern? What ventilatory measurement would be useful in assessing ability to breathe in this situation?

3. A patient admitted for toxic gas inhalation has sustained damage to the airways. When auscultated, the patient exhibits inspiratory "crackles" (a sign of alveolar collapse) throughout most lung fields. The patient's work of breathing is very high. The attending physicians are discussing the possibility of administering synthetic surfactant to the patient's lower airways. Why?

Chapter 4

Ventilation

▷ Points to Remember

- Air is a gas mixture of nitrogen (about 78%) and oxygen (20.93%).
- Barometric pressure at sea level is 760 mm Hg. This value is used for many physiologic gas calculations.
- Atmospheric carbon dioxide pressure is usually considered zero in inspired air.
- Water vapor in the lung has a constant partial pressure of 47 mm Hg (regardless of barometric pressure), which must be subtracted from barometric pressure before calculating other partial pressures in the lung.
- Minute ventilation is the volume of fresh air entering the lung each minute. It is the product of tidal volume and breathing frequency.
- Only part of the minute ventilation ventilates the alveoli. This portion of minute ventilation is called *alveolar ventilation*. The remaining portion ventilates conducting airways and is called *deadspace ventilation*.
- Anatomical deadspace does not change unless an artificial airway is in place or pulmonary anatomy is surgically altered. Hyperinflation (acute or chronic, as in emphysema) increases deadspace because conducting airways dilate, increasing deadspace volume.
- Anatomical deadspace gas at end-inspiration is humidified atmospheric air and at end-expiration is alveolar gas. This gas is inspired at the beginning of the next inspiration.
- Alveolar deadspace is abnormal. It exists when pulmonary blood flow is decreased or absent, as occurs with very low cardiac output or pulmonary embolus.
- Physiological deadspace is the sum of anatomical and alveolar deadspace. It is increased not only by decreased pulmonary blood flow, but also by increased breathing frequency.
- Hyperventilation exists when alveolar ventilation removes more carbon dioxide than is metabolically produced, causing hypocapnia.
- Hypoventilation exists when alveolar ventilation removes less carbon dioxide than is metabolically produced, causing hypercapnia.
- Alveolar ventilation is inversely related to alveolar carbon dioxide partial pressure.
- Increased minute ventilation without a proportionate increase in tidal volume results in increased deadspace ventilation (a high deadspace to tidal volume ratio).

- Deadspace ventilation is increased when pulmonary perfusion is decreased.
- Rapid (tachypnea), shallow (hypopnea) breathing is inefficient ventilation and usually signals respiratory distress.
- Slow (bradypnea), deep (hyperpnea) breathing is the most efficient form of ventilation in terms of percent of minute ventilation used in alveolar ventilation.

▶ The Basics

I. Partial Pressures of Respiratory Gases

1. Match each term on the left with its description on the right:
   _____ Nitrogen
   _____ Oxygen
   _____ Carbon dioxide
   _____ Barometric pressure
   _____ Dalton's law
   _____ Water vapor

   A. Trace gas in air
   B. 760 mm Hg at sea level
   C. Greatest atmospheric partial pressure
   D. Pressure must be subtracted to calculate partial pressures in the lung
   E. Each gas exerts a partial pressure proportional to its concentration
   F. Comprises about 21% of atmospheric air

2. In any geographical location, air pressure is equal to:
   A. 760 mm Hg
   B. The sum of nitrogen and oxygen partial pressures
   C. The sum of nitrogen, oxygen, and carbon dioxide partial pressures
   D. Local barometric pressure

3. In any geographical location, the pressure of inspired air at the carina in spontaneously breathing individuals is equal to:
   A. 760 mm Hg
   B. The sum of nitrogen and oxygen partial pressures
   C. The sum of nitrogen, oxygen, and carbon dioxide partial pressures
   D. Local barometric pressure

4. Water vapor pressure in the lung at any altitude is:
   A. 159 mm Hg
   B. 47 mm Hg
   C. 0.228 mm Hg
   D. 149 mm Hg

II. Ventilation Concepts

5. Minute ventilation is calculated by multiplying the _____ times the _____.

6. A patient has a tidal volume of 450 ml and a respiratory rate of 20 breaths per minute. The calculated minute ventilation is:
   A. 9 L/min
   B. 2.25 L/min
   C. 90 L/min
   D. None of the above

7. If respiratory frequency is known, *alveolar* minute ventilation can be calculated if you also know the:
   A. Minute ventilation
   B. Minute ventilation and tidal volume
   C. Minute ventilation and deadspace volume
   D. Tidal volume

8. Anatomical deadspace is comprised of ventilated airways that do not normally participate in gas exchange with the circulatory system. These airways include the:
   A. Terminal bronchioles and acini
   B. Terminal bronchioles and trachea
   C. Mouth, nose, and respiratory bronchioles
   D. Trachea and respiratory bronchioles

9. Tidal volume is equal to:
   A. The sum of alveolar minute ventilation and deadspace minute ventilation
   B. The sum of alveolar volume and deadspace volume in one breath
   C. Minute ventilation minus deadspace minute ventilation
   D. Deadspace volume minus alveolar volume in one breath

10. Patient A has a deadspace volume of 150 ml, a tidal volume of 450 ml, and a respiratory frequency of 10. Patient B has a deadspace volume of 150 ml, a tidal volume of 350 ml, and a respiratory frequency of 16. Calculate the following physiologic parameters for each patient:

	Patient A	Patient B
A. Minute ventilation	_____	_____
B. Deadspace minute ventilation	_____	_____
C. Alveolar minute ventilation	_____	_____
D. Alveolar ventilation as a percent of minute ventilation	_____	_____
E. Deadspace ventilation as a percent of minute ventilation	_____	_____

11. Partial pressure of carbon dioxide measured at the mouth at the end of expiration (end-tidal carbon dioxide partial pressure) is:
    A. A mixture of partial pressures of anatomical deadspace and alveolar carbon dioxide
    B. Equal to the average partial pressure of carbon dioxide in the alveoli
    C. Equal to the partial pressure of deadspace carbon dioxide at end-inspiration
    D. A mixture of partial pressures of deadspace and atmospheric carbon dioxide

12. A higher-than-normal deadspace volume to tidal volume ratio indicates:
    A. Inefficient ventilation
    B. Low ventilatory energy expenditure
    C. Efficient ventilation
    D. Disproportionately large tidal volumes

13. Hyperventilation exists if clinical findings include:
    A. Rapid shallow breathing
    B. Slow deep breathing
    C. Abnormally high arterial carbon dioxide tension
    D. Abnormally low arterial carbon dioxide tension

14. The definitive index for alveolar ventilation is:
    A. Minute ventilation minus estimated deadspace ventilation
    B. Arterial carbon dioxide tension
    C. Arterial oxygen tension
    D. Tidal volume times breathing frequency

15. If blood flow to a region of alveoli is decreased, the average alveolar partial pressure of carbon dioxide is:
    A. Above normal alveolar carbon dioxide partial pressure
    B. Lower than atmospheric carbon dioxide partial pressure
    C. Below normal
    D. Unchanged from normal

▶ Putting It All Together

1. Patient A has normal conducting airways. Patient B breathes only through a stoma, a surgical opening in the trachea just below the thyroid cartilage. Both patients have identical breathing rates and tidal volumes. Both have similar heights and weights. Comparing these two patients, alveolar ventilation is:
    A. Greater in Patient B
    B. Greater in Patient A
    C. The same in both patients
    D. Not comparable for the two patients with the given information

2. If the inspired air in a dehydrated patient's lungs is drier than normal, oxygen tension is:
    A. Lower than normal
    B. Higher than the atmospheric partial pressure of oxygen
    C. Higher than normal
    D. Equal to the atmospheric partial pressure of oxygen

3. In question 10 in "The Basics" section, which patient has the most efficient ventilation? Why?

4. You begin breathing through a tube 1 meter long. You maintain the same tidal volumes and breathing frequency as before breathing through the tube. Ventilation has changed from normal because now deadspace ventilation is (greater, smaller); mixed expired carbon dioxide concentration is (greater, smaller); alveolar carbon dioxide concentration is (greater, smaller); and alveolar ventilation is (greater, smaller). The ventilatory parameter (other than tidal volume and breathing frequency) unchanged from normal is _____.

5. Mechanical ventilator settings for a patient weighing 200 pounds are tidal volume, 600 ml and breaths per minute, 15. An arterial blood gas obtained on these settings measures arterial carbon dioxide at 45 mm Hg. Calculate the following:
Estimated anatomical deadspace: _____
Minute ventilation: _____
Alveolar ventilation: _____
Deadspace/tidal volume ratio: _____
Alveolar ventilation required to reduce arterial carbon dioxide to 40 mm Hg: _____

Minute ventilation needed for new alveolar ventilation (assuming constant V_D/V_T): _____

6. A carbon dioxide monitor attached to the endotracheal tube of an intubated patient reveals an end-tidal carbon dioxide partial pressure that is 3 mm Hg lower than arterial carbon dioxide analyzed at the same time. This variance:
   A. Is abnormal; end-tidal PCO_2 should be higher than arterial PCO_2
   B. Represents a normal alveolar-arterial PCO_2 gradient
   C. Represents abnormal alveolar deadspace
   D. Is abnormal; the alveolar-arterial PCO_2 gradient is normally greater than 10 mm Hg

7. A patient presents with abnormally high breathing rates and abnormally large tidal volumes. To evaluate this patient's ventilation efficiency, the best information to gather is:
   A. Minute ventilation and breathing frequency
   B. Deadspace/tidal volume ratio and arterial carbon dioxide concentration
   C. Deadspace/tidal volume ratio and arterial oxygen concentration
   D. Minute ventilation and tidal volume

8. A bronchodilator drug is administered to a patient experiencing acute, severe airway constriction and hypercapnia. The drug decreases the abnormally high arterial carbon dioxide levels because:
   A. Minute ventilation increases
   B. Alveolar ventilation increases
   C. Tidal volume increases
   D. Deadspace volume decreases

▷ Cases to Consider

1. A respiratory care practitioner (RCP) is managing the ventilator for a patient totally supported by mechanical breaths. Another bedside caregiver asks the RCP to add a length of tubing between the end of the endotracheal tube and the Y connector of the inspiratory and expiratory limbs of the ventilator tubing to facilitate moving the patient in bed. The respiratory care practitioner states that doing so will result in hypercapnia, since the requested additional tubing has a volume of about 100 ml and the patient's PCO_2 is currently in the normal range. How did the practitioner arrive at this conclusion? Is it possible to honor the request and avoid hypercapnia?

2. A patient with emphysema arrives at the clinic with a complaint of "needing to breathe more and faster than I am used to." Pulmonary function test results indicate that she is maintaining her normal lung volumes and airflows. Breath sounds are clear and diminished, not unusual for emphysematous lungs, but breathing frequency is increased from her baseline. There are no signs of pulmonary infection, such as increased or changed sputum quality or increased white blood cells. An arterial blood gas reveals the patient's normal oxygenation status and an arterial carbon dioxide partial pressure equal to the patient's normal level. The physician, when interviewing the patient, discovers that she has recently made a significant increase in dietary carbohydrates. The physician then asks the clinic nutritionist to instruct the patient on a low-carbohydrate diet. The nutritionist explains to the patient that the primary benefit of a low-carbohydrate diet is lower metabolic carbon dioxide production. Why is the diet change important to this patient and what prompted the physician to ask for the dietary instruction?

3. A patient presents with abnormally low arterial oxygen concentration. Because a low PaO_2 is a ventilatory stimulant, the patient's breathing frequency is 38 breaths per minute and, consequently, arterial carbon dioxide concentration is 34 mm Hg (normal, 40 mm Hg). After one-half hour breathing 100% supplemental oxygen, breathing frequency has slowed to 20 breaths per minute, arterial carbon dioxide is 60 mm Hg, and arterial oxygen concentration remains below normal. The attending RCP states that mechanical ventilatory support may be needed soon. Why?

Chapter 5

Pulmonary Function Measurements

▶ Points to Remember

- Pulmonary function values are classified as normal if the values are within 20% (more or less) of predicted values.
- Severity of pulmonary impairment is based on percent of predicted normal value; age, height, and gender are the main determinants of normal values.
- Residual volume (RV) and any capacity containing RV cannot be directly measured by spirometry.
- Helium dilution, nitrogen washout, and body plethysmography are techniques used to indirectly measure RV and RV-containing capacities.
- Body plethysmography measures total lung volume even in the presence of air trapping.
- RV and functional residual capacity (FRC) are decreased in diseases that increase lung recoil (e.g., fibrotic lung diseases and adult respiratory distress syndrome) and in thoracic cage deformity (e.g., kyphoscoliosis).
- Decreased RV and FRC states are classified as restrictive disease processes.
- RV and FRC are increased by reductions in lung recoil (e.g., emphysema and aging) and by airway obstruction (e.g., bronchospasm and emphysema).
- Increased RV and FRC states are classified as obstructive disease processes.
- Bronchodilator drugs can normalize FRC in reversible bronchospasm but not in passive airway compression, as with emphysema.
- Neuromuscular diseases may exhibit a normal FRC but increased RV because of weak expiratory muscles.
- The hallmark of obstructive pulmonary disease is a reduced expiratory flow rate; the hallmark of restrictive pulmonary disease is reduced lung volumes and capacities.
- Subjects with airway obstruction may have a reduced forced vital capacity (FVC) because of air trapping; or they may have a normal FVC and require longer-than-normal exhalation time.
- The most clinically useful forced expiratory volume measurement is the amount of the FVC exhaled in 1 second (FEV_1).
- Obstructive FEV_1s are low because forced expiratory flow rates are reduced; restrictive and neuromuscular FEV_1s are low because FVCs are reduced.

- The $FEV_1\%$ (FEV_1 divided by FVC) is useful in differentiating restrictive and obstructive diseases. A low FEV_1 and $FEV_1\%$ indicate obstructive impairment. A normal or elevated $FEV_1\%$ with a low FEV_1 indicates a restrictive disorder.
- Peak expiratory flow (PEF) is the highest expiratory flow rate attained during an FVC effort and is useful in assessing gross changes in airway function.
- Maximum voluntary ventilation (MVV) has the greatest variation of all pulmonary function tests; it is about equal to $FEV_1 \times 40$.
- Maximum sustainable ventilation (MSV) is the voluntary hyperventilation sustainable for 10 to 15 minutes; it is equal to about 50% of the MVV in stable COPD patients and about 80% in healthy individuals.
- Tests for small airways disease include frequency dependence of compliance, closing volume, and low-density gas spirometry.

▶ The Basics

I. Static Lung Volumes

1. To be classified in the "normal" range, pulmonary function must be within:
   A. 10% of the predicted value
   B. 20% of the predicted value
   C. 25% of the predicted value
   D. 30% of the predicted value

2. Of the following, the only lung volume that can be measured by *direct* spirometry is:
   A. Residual volume
   B. Functional residual capacity
   C. Vital capacity
   D. Total lung capacity

3. Complete the following table by writing in the "% predicted" range for each degree of impairment.

Degree of impairment	% Predicted
Normal	_____
Mild	_____
Moderate	_____
Severe	_____
Very severe	_____

4. The end-point of the helium dilution FRC test occurs when:
   A. Helium concentration in the lung is lowest
   B. Helium concentration in the spirometer is highest
   C. Helium is eliminated from the spirometer-patient system
   D. Helium concentration is equal throughout the spirometer-patient system

5. The nitrogen washout FRC test is based on the assumption that:
   A. Nitrogen concentration in the lung is normally about 80%
   B. 100% of the oxygen in the lung can be washed out by nitrogen
   C. Nitrogen washout quantifies trapped air volume
   D. Spirometer-lung nitrogen concentrations will equilibrate during the test

6. Body plethysmography is based on Boyle's law, which states that when gas volume and pressure changes occur, initial volume times initial pressure equals:
   A. Final volume times initial pressure
   B. Final volume times final pressure
   C. Initial volume divided by final pressure
   D. Final volume divided by final pressure

7. Results of body plethysmography and helium dilution tests for a patient with early airway collapse will demonstrate:
   A. Equal FRC in both tests
   B. Equal TLC in both tests
   C. Smaller FRC in helium dilution than in plethysmography
   D. The most accurate TLC in helium dilution

8. All of the following are examples of *pulmonary* factors that reduce FRC and RV *except*:
   A. Parenchymal fibrosis
   B. Interstitial edema
   C. Pneumonia
   D. Broken ribs

9. An example of restrictive pulmonary disease is:
   A. Bronchial tumor
   B. Cystic fibrosis
   C. Asthma
   D. Congestive heart failure

10. The *major* pulmonary function characteristic of obstructive pulmonary disease is:
    A. Reduced maximum expiratory flow rate
    B. Increased TLC
    C. Reduced lung volumes and capacities
    D. Low lung compliance

11. On the figure below, complete the labeling and state the average normal values for indicated volumes and capacities.

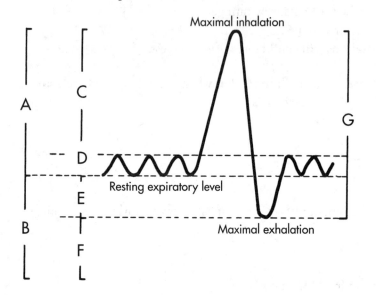

(Art from Scanlan CL, Spearman CB, Sheldon RL: *Egan's fundamentals of respiratory care*, ed 6, St Louis, 1995, Mosby.)

II. Dynamic Pulmonary Mechanics Measurements

12. Results of a series of three FVC maneuvers for a single patient are valid if variance between maneuvers is not greater than:
    A. 10%
    B. 5%
    C. 7%
    D. 15%

13. Compared to FVC results in severely obstructed individuals, slow VC results demonstrate:
    A. Less expiratory time
    B. Greater peak expiratory flow rates
    C. Larger vital capacities
    D. Smaller vital capacities

14. Pulmonary function measurements of purely restrictive impairments include all of the following results *except*:
    A. Decreased FEV_1
    B. Decreased $FEV_1\%$
    C. Decreased FVC
    D. Decreased TLC

15. Pulmonary function measurements of emphysema include all of the following *except*:
    A. Decreased FEV_1
    B. Decreased $FEV_1\%$
    C. Decreased FVC
    D. Decreased TLC

16. The three most common variables used to distinguish between obstructive and restrictive pulmonary function patterns are:
    A. FVC, FEV_1, and $FEV_1\%$
    B. FVC, $FEF_{25\%-75\%}$, and FEV_1
    C. FVC, PEF, and $FEV_1\%$
    D. FVC, FEV_1, and PEF

17. $FEF_{25\%-75\%}$ is an effort (dependent, independent) airway function test.

18. Tests that reflect initial airflows exhaled from large airways include PEF and:
    A. $FEF_{25\%-75\%}$
    B. PIF
    C. $FEV_1\%$
    D. $FEF_{200-1200}$

19. Of the following, the most sensitive test for medium to small airways function is:
    A. $FEF_{200-1200}$
    B. FVC
    C. FEV_1
    D. $FEF_{25\%-75\%}$

20. Label the flow-volume curves in the figure below as "normal," "restrictive," and/or "obstructive."

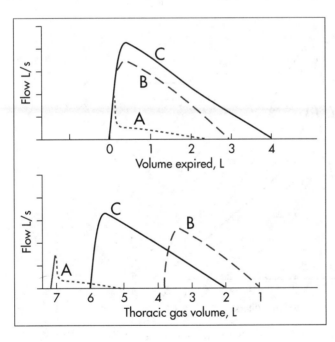

(Art redrawn from Fishman AP: *Assessment of pulmonary function*, New York, 1980, McGraw-Hill.)

21. Maximum sustainable ventilation is a test requiring the subject to sustain maximum voluntary hyperventilation for:
    A. 10 to 15 seconds
    B. 5 to 10 seconds
    C. 5 to 10 minutes
    D. 10 to 15 minutes

III. Tests For Small Airways Disease

22. The standard test against which all other tests of small airway function are measured is:
    A. Frequency dependence of compliance test
    B. Forced expiratory flow between 25% and 75%
    C. Closing volume test
    D. Low-density gas spirometry

23. Reaching onset of phase IV in single-breath nitrogen elimination earlier than normal indicates:
    A. Basal airway closure later in exhaled vital capacity
    B. An increased closing volume
    C. Closing volume is 10% to 20%
    D. Basal alveoli are contributing to expiratory gas flow

24. Low-density gas spirometry compares two types of flow-volume curves. One type is done while breathing room air and the other type is done while breathing:
    A. 80% nitrogen and 20% oxygen
    B. 100% oxygen
    C. 80% helium and 20% oxygen
    D. 80% oxygen and 20% helium

25. On the graph below, indicate the points of volume isoflow and V_{max50}.

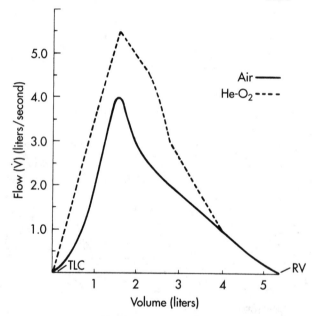

(Art from Ruppel G: *Manual of pulmonary function testing*, ed 6, St Louis, 1994, Mosby.)

▶ Putting It All Together

1. A nitrogen washout test yields the following information: volume of expired gas, 22,850 ml and % N_2, 6%. The calculated FRC is:
   A. 1371 ml
   B. 4570 ml
   C. 1727 ml
   D. 1097 ml

2. The nitrogen washout test above was performed on an average adult male. Without further data, the test results alone are indicative of:
   A. A reduced FRC
   B. An increased FRC
   C. Air trapping
   D. Reduced thoracic gas volume

3. A long-term ventilator patient with an endotracheal tube still in place is being evaluated for possible removal of the tube. By using a special patient-spirometer interface, an FVC is performed to determine "weanability" from the ventilator. The test value that will be most different from breathing without the endotracheal tube in place is:
   A. FEV_1
   B. $FEF_{25\%-75\%}$
   C. $FEF_{50\%}$
   D. $FEF_{75\%}$

4. Of the three spirometric values, FVC, FEV_1, and $FEV_1\%$, obstructive and restrictive lung diseases are distinguished from each other primarily by $FEV_1\%$. Why?

5. Guillain-Barré is a debilitating neuromuscular disease that may affect the ventilatory muscles. Performing FVC maneuvers is important in monitoring progression of this disease because:
   A. The maneuvers require little patient effort, which is impaired in this disease
   B. A change in FRC volume is extrapolated from the results
   C. It is an effort-dependent test, reflecting ventilatory strength
   D. A reduction in TLC can be measured

6. A patient with an esophageal balloon in place is noted to have a dynamic-to-static compliance ratio significantly below normal. Even though the patient's spirometric lung volumes and expiratory flows are normal, possible diagnoses based on this test will include:
   A. Asthma
   B. Pulmonary fibrosis
   C. Pulmonary sarcoidosis
   D. Pleuritis

7. Emphysema causes an increase in the volume of isoflow in the low-density gas spirometry test. This occurs because:
   A. Dynamic airway compression occurs later in an FVC maneuver
   B. Laminar flow develops earlier in an FVC maneuver
   C. Expiratory flow changes from laminar to turbulent
   D. The helium-oxygen FVC is smaller than the room air FVC

8. If, during a plethysmography test, the body box airtight seal is disrupted, FRC calculation will be different than a calculation done under airtight conditions because:
   A. Mouthpiece occlusion pressure during inspiration will be lower
   B. Initial mouth pressure will be greater
   C. Body box pressure during inspiration will be greater
   D. There will be a smaller change in body box pressure during inspiration

▶ Cases to Consider

1. As the clinic educator for pulmonary patients, you have received a request from one of the family practice physicians to review a patient's recent spirometry results with him. The patient has just been given a diagnosis of pulmonary disease and needs an understanding of what his disease "is all about." He is a long-term smoker who has become progressively short of breath with exertion over the past 2 to 3 years. The recent spirometry test revealed subnormal values for FVC (75% of predicted), FEV_1 (50% of predicted), and FEV_1% (50% of predicted). Spirometry had also been performed after administration of a bronchodilator. Changes in FVC, FEV_1, and FEV_1% were less than 15% and were considered insignificant responses to the bronchodilator. To prepare for the educational session with this patient, you must decide what type of lung disease is reflected in the spirometric values. Is restrictive or obstructive lung disease present? What diagnostic test could further support your assessment?

2. The clinical summary of a 48-year-old patient has been sent for your review as the supervisor of a pulmonary function laboratory. The patient's history and physical include current treatment for pulmonary sarcoidosis. During recent clinic visits, peak flow values (using a simple peak flowmeter) were documented as normal to greater than normal. The treating physician has requested that this patient's pulmonary disease be verified as primarily obstructive or restrictive by the pulmonary function laboratory using simple spirometry. What is your pulmonary function test of choice and why?

Chapter 6

Pulmonary Blood Flow

▷ Points to Remember

- The pump for systemic circulation is the left ventricle; the right ventricle serves the pulmonary circulation.
- Pulmonary veins and venules carry oxygenated blood and pulmonary arteries and arterioles carry deoxygenated blood; this is opposite from the systemic circulation.
- Approximately half of the deoxygenated systemic bronchial blood dilutes the oxygen concentration of oxygenated blood returning to the left ventricle, resulting in about 2% shunt.
- The pulmonary circulation is a low-resistance, low-pressure system; the systemic circulation is a high-resistance, high-pressure system. The same cardiac output passes through both circulations.
- Communicating with strategically placed openings along the Swan-Ganz pulmonary artery catheter, transducers directly measure right atrial pressure (RAP) or central venous pressure (CVP) and pulmonary artery pressure (PAP).
- When the balloon on the distal end of the Swan-Ganz catheter is inflated to occlude the pulmonary artery, the pressure measured at the catheter tip (pulmonary capillary wedge pressure [PCWP]) reflects the left atrial pressure (also known as left ventricular filling pressure or left ventricular preload).
- Blood drawn from the Swan-Ganz catheter channel communicating with the right atrium (the *proximal* channel) is deoxygenated, but clinically acceptable *mixed venous* samples must be drawn from the *distal* channel communicating with the pulmonary artery.
- Tissue oxygen consumption is evaluated by comparing arterial oxygen content with mixed venous oxygen content.
- Pulmonary vascular resistance (PVR) is the resistance against which the right ventricle pumps; systemic vascular resistance (SVR) must be overcome by the left ventricle.
- Alveolar capillaries are in intimate contact with alveolar walls and are compressed by alveolar inflation, increasing pulmonary vascular resistance during inspiration.
- Total PVR is the composite of alveolar and extraalveolar vessel resistances and is lowest at FRC. Lung volumes above and below FRC increase PVR.

- Increased pulmonary vascular pressure decreases PVR because of vascular distension and recruitment of collapsed capillaries.
- Nitric oxide (NO) is synthesized by vessel endothelial cells. Increased NO causes vasodilation and decreased PVR.
- Excessive NO levels are responsible for massive vasodilation and hypotension in septic shock.
- Hypoxic pulmonary vasoconstriction increases PVR and, conversely, improved oxygenation will decrease PVR in hypoxic individuals.
- Zone I blood flow (normally non-existent in pulmonary circulation) has no blood flow due to alveolar compression of capillaries.
- In zone II blood flow, alveolar pressure exceeds venous pressure but not arterial pressure, causing intermittent flow through alveolar capillaries.
- In zone III blood flow, arterial and venous pressures exceed alveolar pressures. This zone has the greatest blood flow.
- Because of increased compliance in basilar alveoli, ventilation is greatest in the lung bases.
- Deadspace refers to the ventilation of alveoli with no perfusion.
- Shunt refers to perfusion of alveoli with no ventilation.
- Ventilation-perfusion ratios normally range from high in lung apices to low in lung bases. The overall ventilation-perfusion ratio in the normal resting lung is 0.8.
- Pulmonary edema is caused by increased hydrostatic pressure, increased capillary permeability, decreased plasma oncotic pressure, and insufficient lymphatic drainage.

▶ The Basics

I. Pulmonary Vasculature

1. Number the following circulatory structures sequentially, starting with the first structure deoxygenated blood encounters when returning to the heart.
   _____ Systemic arterioles
   _____ Left ventricle
   _____ Systemic arteries
   _____ Right atrium
   _____ Pulmonary artery
   _____ Pulmonary veins
   _____ Pulmonic valve
   _____ Mitral valve
   _____ Pulmonary capillaries

2. Of the vessels below, oxygenated blood passing by an alveolus initially encounters the:
   A. Pulmonary arteriole
   B. Pulmonary artery
   C. Pulmonary venule
   D. Pulmonary vein

II. Pulmonary and Systemic Pressures

3. Pulmonary circulation pulse pressure:
   A. Is smaller than systemic pulse pressure
   B. Results in more continuous blood flow compared to systemic flow
   C. Results in highly pulsatile flow, compared to systemic flow
   D. Remains minimally pulsatile during ventilation

4. Match the pulmonary artery catheter part on the left with its intended use(s) on the right. (Note: Some parts may have more than one use.)

   _____ Balloon
   _____ Thermistor
   _____ Proximal lumen
   _____ Distal lumen

   A. Used to access true mixed venous blood
   B. Used to calculate cardiac output
   C. Used to measure CVP
   D. Used to measure PAP
   E. Used to measure PCWP
   F. Used to flow-direct catheter during insertion
   G. Used to measure pulmonary venous pressure

5. PCWP reflects all of the following *except*:
   A. Left ventricular preload
   B. Left ventricular end-diastolic pressure
   C. Pulmonary venous pressure
   D. Pulmonary artery pressure

6. The proximal channel of the Swan-Ganz catheter is used to assess all of the following *except*:
   A. Right atrial pressure
   B. Pulmonary artery pressure
   C. Central venous pressure
   D. Right ventricular preload

7. Excessively high PCWP consistently indicates:
   A. Left ventricular failure
   B. Hypervolemia
   C. Pulmonary capillary engorgement
   D. Mitral valve stenosis

8. A Swan-Ganz thermistor senses a rapid temperature change toward normal after cool fluid bolus injection; this indicates:
   A. High cardiac output
   B. Low pulmonary artery pressure
   C. Low cardiac output
   D. High pulmonary vascular resistance

III. Pulmonary Vascular Resistance

9. Passive and active factors affect pulmonary vascular resistance. In the list below, specify whether each factor is active (A) or passive (P).
   _____ Pulmonary capillary recruitment
   _____ Alveolar pressure
   _____ Left ventricular failure
   _____ Endogenous nitric oxide
   _____ Low P_AO_2
   _____ Arterial pH less than 7.30
   _____ Systemic blood loss

10. During lung inflation, extraalveolar vessels:
    A. Are compressed by alveolar pressure
    B. Are dilated by increased pulmonary artery pressure
    C. Are dilated by alveolar recoil
    D. Add to overall pulmonary vascular resistance

11. All of the following *decrease* pulmonary vascular resistance *except*:
    A. Decreased cardiac output
    B. Increased pulmonary blood volume
    C. Left ventricular failure
    D. Increased nitric oxide levels

12. An important effect of generalized hypoxemia is:
    A. Systemic vasodilation
    B. Hypoxic pulmonary vasodilation
    C. Decreased pulmonary vascular resistance
    D. Diversion of blood to poorly oxygenated alveoli

13. Hypoxic pulmonary vasoconstriction physiologic benefits include:
    A. Diverting blood to poorly ventilated areas of the lung
    B. Elevation of left atrial pressure
    C. Improved mixing of blood from ventilated and non-ventilated areas
    D. An improved match between blood flow and ventilation

14. Release of nitric oxide is known to be induced by all of the following *except*:
    A. cNOS production in physical exercise
    B. Sympathetic neurogenic stimulation
    C. Endothelial stretching
    D. iNOS production in septicemia

IV. Distribution of Pulmonary Blood Flow

15. Zone I pulmonary blood flow occurs whenever:
    A. Alveolar pressure exceeds arterial and venous blood pressures
    B. Blood circulates through apical capillaries
    C. Alveolar pressure exceeds pulmonary venous pressure
    D. Flow through pulmonary capillaries becomes intermittent

16. Zone II blood flow is:
    A. Proportional to arterial-venous pressure gradients
    B. Determined by the difference between arterial and alveolar pressure
    C. Dependent on venous capillary pressure
    D. Determined by venous rate of flow

17. Blood flow in zone III is:
    A. Gravity independent
    B. Normally affected by alveolar pressure
    C. Proportional to the alveolar-venous pressure gradient
    D. Determined by the arterial-venous pressure gradient

18. A low ventilation-perfusion ratio is typical of:
    A. A deadspace-like situation
    B. Ventilation-perfusion matching in the apices
    C. Basilar ventilation and perfusion
    D. The normal response to exercise

V. Liquid Movement Across the Alveolar-Capillary Membrane

19. As the concentration of protein molecules increases in blood plasma:
    A. Water molecules are "pulled" into the vessels
    B. Plasma osmotic pressure decreases
    C. Plasma oncotic pressure decreases
    D. Fluid is "pushed out" of the vessels

20. Net mean filtration pressure between capillaries and interstitial spaces:
    A. Causes a continuous flow from interstitial spaces into capillaries
    B. Is about 1 mm Hg from interstitial spaces into capillaries
    C. Favors fluid movement out of capillaries into interstitial spaces
    D. Is the result of 29 mm Hg of hydrostatic pressure

21. Causes of pulmonary edema *do not* include:
    A. Increased plasma oncotic pressure
    B. Increased hydrostatic pressure
    C. Increased capillary permeability
    D. Insufficient lymphatic drainage

22. In cardiogenic pulmonary edema, fluid accumulates in interstitial spaces primarily because of:
    A. Increased hydrostatic pressure
    B. Increased capillary permeability
    C. Decreased plasma oncotic pressure
    D. Increased fluid oncotic pressure

23. Interstitial fluid accumulation secondary to mitral valve stenosis is caused by:
    A. Increased capillary permeability
    B. Decreased plasma oncotic pressure
    C. Increased hydrostatic pressure
    D. Decreased interstitial oncotic pressure

▶ Putting It All Together

1. A patient who has a Swan-Ganz catheter in place has become very restless and is moving around in bed continuously. To update the patient's hemodynamic status, a PCWP measurement is attempted, but the waveform during the wedge procedure does not change. It remains identical to the PA waveform. Considering this information, possible causes include:
   A. Disconnection of the transducer
   B. Migration of the distal end of the catheter to the right ventricle
   C. Kinking and occlusion of the external portion of the catheter
   D. Loss of the balloon's "wedge" position in the pulmonary artery

2. A septicemic patient is exhibiting an abnormally low PVR and a normal PCWP. This is consistent with:
   A. Hypervolemia
   B. Cardiogenic pulmonary edema
   C. Hypovolemia
   D. High nitric oxide levels

3. High positive end-expiratory pressure and extended inspiratory time may cause an elevated PVR. This occurs because:
   A. Shunt is increased
   B. Zone I lung volume is increased
   C. Zone III lung volume is increased
   D. Extraalveolar vessels have collapsed

4. A hypovolemic patient is given intravenous fluid. PVR before the fluid infusion was above normal and PAP was below normal. After the fluid infusion, PVR dropped and PAP rose. Why?

5. High inspiratory pressures during positive-pressure ventilation can lead to alveolar hyperdistension and alveolar capillary compression. This can cause abnormal ventilation-perfusion in some lung fields. This condition is known as:
   A. Shunt-like effect
   B. Low ventilation-perfusion ratio
   C. Deadspace-like effect
   D. Zone III blood flow and ventilation

6. Causes for an abnormally high PAP accompanying an abnormally high PCWP in a hypoxic patient include:
   A. Hypovolemia and pulmonary vasoconstriction
   B. Hypovolemia and mitral valve stenosis
   C. Left ventricular failure and pulmonary vasoconstriction
   D. Hypervolemia and low left ventricular preload

7. Cardiogenic pulmonary edema is being treated with diuretics. A beneficial outcome of diuretic therapy is:
   A. Capillary recruitment and distension
   B. Decreased pulmonary blood volume
   C. Decreased PVR
   D. Increased PAP

8. If a malpositioned pulmonary artery catheter resides in the pulmonary artery but cannot be adjusted to obtain a PCWP, the best estimation for this pressure (if PVR is normal) is:
   A. Systolic pulmonary artery pressure
   B. Central venous pressure
   C. Mean pulmonary artery pressure
   D. Diastolic pulmonary artery pressure

9. A hypoxemic, hypervolemic patient with congestive heart failure has been placed on a high concentration of oxygen. Another therapy that would benefit this patient is administering:
   A. Vasodilators
   B. Inotropic agents
   C. Diuretics
   D. Fluid boluses

▶ Cases to Consider

1. You are a critical care respiratory therapist assisting in the management of a mechanically ventilated 65-year-old male patient. The patient was admitted directly to the intensive care unit (ICU) after arriving at an outpatient clinic in severe respiratory distress. Shortly after admission to the ICU, breath sounds were wheezy with diffuse inspiratory crackles throughout the lungs and arterial blood gases revealed impending respiratory failure. The patient was intubated and placed on mechanical ventilation. Because the patient had a history of congestive heart failure and low systemic blood pressures, a Swan-Ganz catheter was placed to monitor the patient's hemodynamic status. When reviewing your first cardiac output measurement for this individual, you make the following observations: the PAP is elevated above normal; the PCWP is elevated above normal; the PAP-PCWP difference is normal; cardiac output is low; systemic blood pressure is below normal; and PVR is low, but within normal limits. Another practitioner just coming on shift questions you regarding the cause of the abnormal hemodynamic values and the factors precipitating the need for mechanical ventilation. What is your response?

2. One day later, the patient in the case above has stabilized and you are decreasing the ventilatory support and supplemental oxygen. While the patient is still on the ventilator and still has the Swan-Ganz catheter in place, the attending physician orders a cardiac output measurement and arterial blood gas analysis to be done in 1 hour. As the attending respiratory care practitioner, you note that, during the ensuing hour, the patient's total breathing frequency and work of breathing are increased and breath sounds are decreased from previous assessments. You perform the cardiac output measurement and draw the arterial blood gas sample and, while awaiting the results of both procedures, you suction the patient's endotracheal tube, extracting a large mucous plug from the airway. Immediately, work of breathing and breathing frequency return to normal and good air exchange is auscultated throughout all lung fields. The physician reviewing the diagnostic results comments on the abnormally high PAP and PVR in the presence of a normal PCWP. The arterial blood gas reveals hypoxemia. You tell the physician about suctioning the patient and state that a second cardiac output and arterial blood gas done in about a 30 minutes will probably demonstrate normal hemodynamic and arterial blood gas results. How can your comments be justified?

3. An ICU patient with a history of emphysema and chronic hypoxemia has a pulmonary artery catheter in place. The patient's baseline hemodynamic pressures include a PCWP that is normal and PAP and CVP values that are above normal. The patient's chest x-ray is interpreted as chronic hyperinflation and enlarged right side of the heart. An echocardiography evaluating cardiac dynamics shows subnormal right ventricular ejection volumes. A medical student asks for your assessment of the etiology of this patient's hemodynamic pressures and enlarged right heart. What is your response?

Chapter 7

Gas Diffusion

▷ Points to Remember

- Diffusion is net molecular movement from high partial pressure to low partial pressure and is the mechanism for gas movement in terminal airways and alveoli.
- Gas transfer across the alveolar-capillary (a-c) membrane occurs at different rates depending on individual gas partial pressure gradients.
- Alveolar air pressure at sea level contains about 100 mm Hg oxygen, 47 mm Hg water vapor, and 40 mm Hg carbon dioxide.
- With a normal value of 0.8, the respiratory exchange ratio (R) represents the exchange of 200 ml/minute of capillary carbon dioxide across the a-c membrane for 250 ml/minute of alveolar oxygen.
- The ideal alveolar air equation accounts for the effects of R on P_AO_2:
  $P_AO_2 = P_IO_2 - P_AO_2 [F_IO_2 + (1 - F_IO_2)/R]$
- Gas diffusion across the a-c membrane is directly proportional to increases in membrane surface area, gas solubility, and the diffusion pressure gradient.
- Diffusion across the a-c membrane is inversely proportional to increases in membrane thickness.
- Alveolar-capillary membrane defects limit oxygen diffusion but do not limit carbon dioxide diffusion.
- Equilibrium between capillary and alveolar oxygen pressures normally occurs in 0.25 second, which is one third of the time it takes the blood to travel through the capillary when the body is at rest.
- Oxygen diffusion across the a-c membrane is normally affected by blood flow rate (perfusion limited).
- Factors thickening the a-c membrane generally do not prevent equilibrium between alveolar and capillary PO_2 except during exercise, which is when capillary blood transit time decreases.
- Because blood takes up carbon monoxide more rapidly than it can diffuse across the a-c membrane, carbon monoxide is useful as a test gas to assess a-c membrane diffusion capacity.

▶ The Basics

I. Diffusion of Respiratory Gases

1. On the illustration below indicate the following:
   A. The gas that is represented by each arrow
   B. The alveolar partial pressure of each gas at sea level
   C. The normal volume of diffusion for each gas in ml/minute

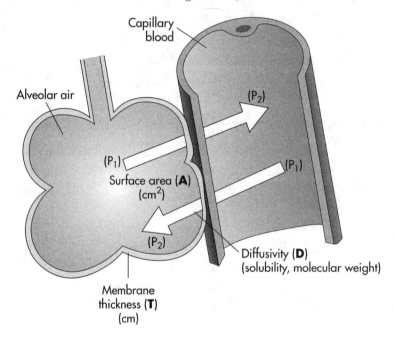

2. Select the statement below that is *not true* about gas diffusion.
   A. Each gas in a mixture diffuses according to the overall mixture's pressure gradient.
   B. Diffusion continues until equilibrium is reached.
   C. Diffusion is the mechanism for gas movement in the terminal bronchioles.
   D. Diffusion represents net movement from high pressure to low pressure.

3. According to the alveolar air equation, all other factors remaining constant, P_AO_2:
   A. Increases as P_ACO_2 increases
   B. Increases as P_IO_2 increases
   C. Decreases as the respiratory exchange ratio increases
   D. Decreases as inspired nitrogen decreases

4. Match the value on the left with the appropriate normal sea level partial pressure or pressure gradient on the right:

   ──── 0 mm Hg   A. Carbon dioxide a-c diffusion gradient
   ──── 6 mm Hg   B. Oxygen partial pressure in inspired air
   ──── 40 mm Hg   C. Alveolar carbon dioxide partial pressure
   ──── 47 mm Hg   D. Capillary carbon dioxide partial pressure
   ──── 46 mm Hg   E. Alveolar oxygen partial pressure
   ──── 60 mm Hg   F. Oxygen a-c diffusion gradient
   ──── 100 mm Hg   G. Carbon dioxide partial pressure in inspired air
   ──── 160 mm Hg   H. Alveolar water vapor partial pressure

5. The normal respiratory exchange ratio is about 0.8. This represents an:
   A. Oxygen-to-carbon dioxide diffusion ratio of 200:250
   B. 80% replacement of oxygen in the alveolus by carbon dioxide
   C. 80% replacement of carbon dioxide in the capillary by oxygen
   D. 80% increase in alveolar nitrogen in response to oxygen's decrease

6. According to Fick's law, the rate of gas diffusion is:
   A. Directly proportional to diffusion path distance
   B. Inversely proportional to membrane surface area available for diffusion
   C. Inversely proportional to membrane thickness
   D. Inversely proportional to the diffusion pressure gradient

7. The diffusion rate for carbon dioxide in a:
   A. Gas mixture is greater than the oxygen diffusion rate
   B. Gas mixture equals the oxygen diffusion rate
   C. Liquid is greater than the oxygen diffusion rate
   D. Liquid equals the oxygen diffusion rate

II. Limitations of Oxygen Diffusion

8. At rest, the amount of time normally required for equilibrium between alveolar and capillary oxygen is:
   A. 0.75 second
   B. One-third the blood travel time in the pulmonary capillary
   C. One-fourth the blood travel time in the pulmonary capillary
   D. 0.5 second

9. Under normal conditions, the oxygen diffusion rate changes during pulmonary capillary transit time because:
   A. Of significant variations in a-c membrane thickness
   B. Blood flow rate decreases during transit time
   C. Blood flow rate increases during transit time
   D. The a-c diffusion gradient narrows as equilibrium approaches

10. Examples of diffusion limitations include all of the following *except*:
    A. Thickened a-c membranes
    B. Low cardiac output
    C. Interstitial edema
    D. Side-by-side red blood cell flow

11. Oxygen transfer across the a-c membrane:
    A. May occur slowly at high altitudes when PO_2 is low
    B. Is not normally perfusion limited
    C. Normally does not reach equilibrium between alveoli and blood with increased cardiac output
    D. Occurs at a constant rate during transit time

12. Carbon monoxide is used for testing diffusion defects in the a-c membrane because:
    A. Normally, equilibrium across the membrane is reached quickly
    B. Changes in cardiac output affect the rate of gas uptake
    C. It is strictly diffusion limited
    D. Its transfer rate is greater than the capillary blood absorption rate

13. Reasons for using nitrous oxide in testing pulmonary blood flow include all of the following *except* that:
    A. Normally, equilibrium across the a-c membrane is reached quickly
    B. Changes in cardiac output affect the rate of gas uptake
    C. It is diffusion limited
    D. Its transfer rate is greater than the capillary blood absorption rate

14. In the two figures that follow, assume that the number of arrows crossing the a-c membrane represents two different rates of gas transfer. Equilibrium between gas and blood is reached in figure "A" at the a-c arrow furthest right but is not reached in figure "B." State whether each is a depiction of perfusion or diffusion limitation.

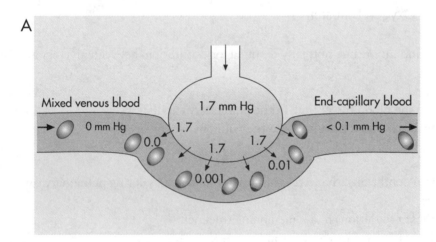

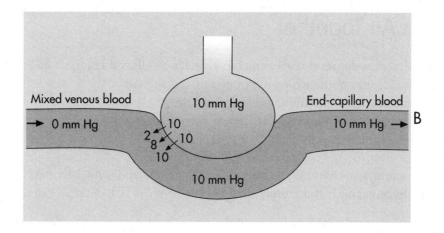

15. In emphysema, reductions in functional gas exchange surface area are caused by all of the following *except*:
    A. Thickened a-c membrane
    B. Destruction of functional gas exchange surface area
    C. Reduced alveolar surface area
    D. Reduced capillary membrane area

III. Measuring Diffusion Capacity

16. Carbon monoxide diffusion capacity ($D_L CO$) normally increases:
    A. After the first 20 years of life
    B. With high lung volumes
    C. In standing body position
    D. In anemic blood conditions

17. For the diffusion capacity defects below, label each as an example of increased diffusion path distance ("P"), decreased diffusion surface area ("S"), decreased uptake by red blood cells ("U"), or ventilation-perfusion mismatch ("M").
    _____ Anemia
    _____ Interstitial fibrosis
    _____ Engorged capillaries
    _____ High carbon monoxide blood levels
    _____ Destruction of alveolar-capillary bed
    _____ Regional atelectasis
    _____ Pulmonary embolus
    _____ Lobar pneumonia

18. An example of abnormally low $D_L CO$ caused by decreased diffusion surface area is:
    A. High carbon monoxide levels secondary to smoking
    B. Alveolar interstitial fibrosis
    C. Abnormally low hemoglobin levels
    D. Reduced capillary blood flow secondary to pulmonary embolus

▶ Putting It All Together

1. Alveolar-capillary gas diffusion is abnormal in alveolar-capillary membrane defects because:
   A. Carbon dioxide may not reach equilibrium during exercise
   B. Oxygen may not reach equilibrium during exercise
   C. Carbon dioxide diffuses more rapidly than oxygen in gases
   D. Oxygen diffuses more rapidly than carbon dioxide in fluids

2. Patients with emphysema exhibit premature airway collapse and some become "CO_2 retainers" (i.e., develop hypercapnia); at atmospheric F_IO_2, the alveolar PO_2 decreases in CO_2 retention because:
   A. P_AH_2O decreases
   B. P_AN_2 decreases
   C. N_2 displaces O_2
   D. CO_2 displaces O_2

3. Administering fluid to a severely dehydrated, hypotensive patient improves diffusion capacity because:
   A. Diffusion surface area is increased
   B. The low ventilation-perfusion ratio is corrected
   C. Red blood cell uptake is improved
   D. Diffusion path distance is decreased

4. Providing positive-pressure ventilatory support to a patient who is hypoventilating and unconscious improves diffusion capacity because:
   A. The diffusion surface area is increased
   B. The low ventilation-perfusion ratio is corrected
   C. Red blood cell uptake ability is improved
   D. The diffusion path distance is decreased

5. We give patients with retained secretions humidified gas to breathe, improving their ability to expectorate and open previously plugged airways. Opening these airways improves diffusion capacity because:
   A. The diffusion surface area is increased
   B. The low ventilation-perfusion ratio is corrected
   C. Red blood cell uptake is improved
   D. The diffusion path distance is decreased

6. Which test gas should be used to evaluate the lung's diffusion capacity when a tumor is compressing a pulmonary artery? Why?

7. Diffusion capacity increases toward normal after a hypervolemic patient with congestive left heart failure is given diuretic therapy. This improvement occurs because:
   A. The diffusion surface area is increased
   B. The low ventilation-perfusion ratio is corrected
   C. Red blood cell uptake is improved
   D. The diffusion path distance is decreased

8. A D_LCO test result shows abnormally low diffusion for a patient with chronic hyperinflation, a significant smoking history, and dependence on supplemental oxygen. The clinical picture indicates the low diffusion rate is due to:
   A. The decreased diffusion surface area
   B. A low ventilation-perfusion ratio
   C. Decreased red blood cell uptake
   D. Increased diffusion path distance

▶ Cases to Consider

1. As the respiratory care practitioner caring for an elderly post-operative hip repair patient, you are being consulted by a physical therapist regarding the patient's ability to ambulate. With a portable pulse oximeter, you note the patient's oxygen saturation to be significantly below normal on room air. The patient is still on 2 liters of oxygen by nasal cannula since surgery 4 days earlier and is only now starting ambulation because of poor pain control. The patient's medical history is negative for any pulmonary or cardiac disease or treatment. The post-operative course includes: inability to wean off supplemental oxygen; immobility for about 96 hours; below normal inspiratory volumes with incentive spirometry; and breath sounds exhibiting bilateral inspiratory crackles. Without the benefit of D_LCO test results, what is your assumption about the patient's diffusion capacity? What is the reason for any diffusion abnormalities? What corrective actions can be taken?

2. You are a respiratory care practitioner assisting a pulmonologist to perform routine annual health appraisals on-site at a large coal mining facility. A worker appears for her appointment with a chief complaint of "tiredness and lack of energy." You note that her spirometry results are consistent with restrictive lung disease. Resting oxygen hemoglobin saturation on room air is normal. A pulmonary stress test indicates sub-optimal oxygenation during exercise. Breath sounds include bilateral fine inspiratory crackles that are present before, during, and after exercise. The pulmonologist asks if you believe a follow-up appointment for a D_LCO test at the pulmonary clinic is indicated. What D_LCO results would you expect and why?

Chapter 8
Oxygen Equilibrium and Transport

▷ Points to Remember

- Ninety-eight percent of the oxygen carried in the blood is bound to hemoglobin.
- Oxygen dissolved in the blood exerts a partial gas pressure (PO_2) and determines the rate and direction of diffusion and the extent to which oxygen binds to hemoglobin.
- Small changes in PO_2 below 60 mm Hg produce large changes in oxygen content and hemoglobin saturation.
- Changes in PO_2 above 60 mm Hg produce minimal changes in oxygen content.
- Decreased pH and increased PCO_2, temperature, and 2,3-DPG shift the oxyhemoglobin equilibrium curve to the right, reflecting a decrease in oxygen's affinity for hemoglobin. Opposite changes shift the curve to the left.
- Decreased hemoglobin affinity for oxygen increases plasma PO_2 and promotes oxygen diffusion to tissues.
- Cardiac output and arterial oxygen content determine the rate of oxygen transport to the tissues.
- The normal tissue oxygen extraction ratio is 25% and increases with exercise, low blood flow, and anemia.
- Five ml/dl or more of deoxygenated hemoglobin in capillary blood produces cyanosis..
- Hypoxia can exist without cyanosis in individuals with severe anemia or carbon monoxide poisoning; conversely, normal blood oxygen content can exist in the presence of cyanosis in polycythemic persons.
- Fetal hemoglobin's high oxygen affinity allows it to carry adequate amounts of oxygen despite a low PO_2.
- Methemoglobinemia causes irreversible binding of oxygen with hemoglobin.
- Deoxygenation in sickle cell anemia causes the red blood cell shape to change, resulting in clumping and vascular occlusions.

▷ The Basics

I. Carrying Oxygen in Blood

1. Dissolved plasma oxygen content is calculated by multiplying arterial oxygen tension by:
   A. The amount of oxygen dissolving in 100 ml plasma
   B. 0.0003
   C. 0.03
   D. The amount of oxygen dissolving in 10 ml plasma

2. Dissolved oxygen content in normal plasma with a PO_2 of 80 mm Hg is:
   A. 2.4 ml/dl
   B. 0.024 ml/dl
   C. 0.24 ml/dl
   D. 24 ml/dl

3. At a PO_2 of 100 mm Hg in normal whole blood, oxygen bound to hemoglobin is approximately:
   A. 0.3 ml/dl
   B. 2 ml/dl
   C. 10 ml/dl
   D. 20 ml/dl

4. Calculate oxygen delivery to the tissues of a patient with a cardiac output of 4 L/min and a normal hemoglobin oxygen content.

5. In the preceding question, is oxygen delivery adequate for resting tissue oxygen uptake?

6. A single oxygenated hemoglobin molecule tends to combine with:
   A. 2 oxygen molecules
   B. 4 oxygen molecules
   C. 6 oxygen molecules
   D. 8 oxygen molecules

7. A deoxygenated hemoglobin molecule carries:
   A. No oxygen molecules
   B. 1 oxygen molecule
   C. 2 oxygen molecules
   D. 4 oxygen molecules

8. A normal PO_2 of 100 mm Hg corresponds with an arterial oxygen saturation of approximately:
   A. 100%
   B. 98%
   C. 97%
   D. 96%

9. Mixed venous oxygen partial pressure of 40 mm Hg corresponds with a mixed venous oxygen saturation of:
   A. 90%
   B. 85%
   C. 80%
   D. 75%

10. What is the general formula for calculating total oxygen content in blood (oxygen bound to hemoglobin and dissolved in plasma)?

11. If 13 grams of normal hemoglobin is 89% saturated with oxygen, the hemoglobin oxygen content is:
    A. 17.4 ml/dl
    B. 15.5 ml/dl
    C. 11.6 ml/dl
    D. 14.6 ml/dl

12. To construct the oxyhemoglobin curve, _____ is plotted on the vertical axis and _____ on the horizontal axis.

13. Between 10 and 40 mm Hg PO_2 on the oxyhemoglobin curve:
    A. Oxygen content changes little for each unit of change in PO_2
    B. Oxygen is normally unloading from hemoglobin
    C. A safety margin exists for oxygen content as PaO_2 decreases
    D. Oxygen is normally loading on hemoglobin

14. The percent of arterial oxygen content normally released from arterial hemoglobin to the tissues is:
    A. 15%
    B. 20%
    C. 25%
    D. 40%

15. A high P_{50} means that:
    A. More than 50 mm Hg PO_2 is required to saturate 50% of hemoglobin
    B. Less than 50 mm Hg PO_2 is required to saturate 50% of hemoglobin
    C. More oxygen is loaded on hemoglobin than at a normal P_{50}
    D. Hemoglobin affinity for oxygen is advantageous for tissue oxygenation

16. On the top graph on p. 61, mark the points on the oxyhemoglobin curve that intersect with PO_2s of 20, 60, and 100 mm Hg. Then, using the "oxygen content" axis, estimate the change in oxygen content as PO_2 increases 40 mm Hg from 20 to 60 mm Hg and from 60 to 100 mm Hg.

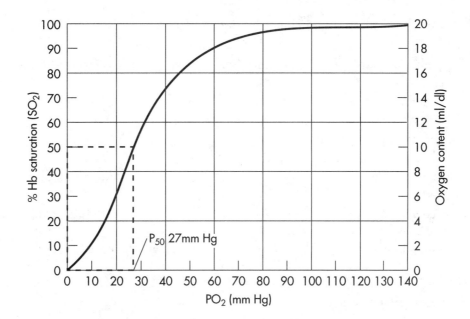

17. On the graph below, draw oxyhemoglobin curves representing right and left shifts and label each curve with the factors that cause its deviation from normal.

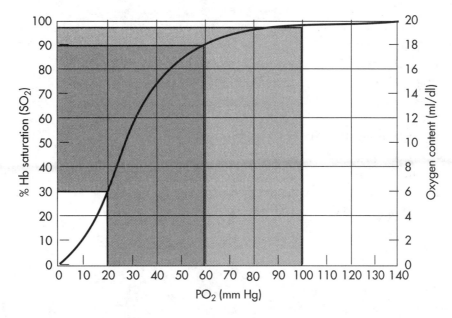

18. A right shift of the oxyhemoglobin curve (increases, decreases) oxygen delivery to the tissues by (increasing, decreasing) plasma PO_2. A left shift in the curve (increases, decreases) hemoglobin's affinity for oxygen and results in (increased, decreased) plasma PO_2.

II. Calculating Oxygen Contents and Tissue Extraction Ratio

19. Place the appropriate letter of the approximate normal value on the right next to the appropriate description on the left.

    _____ Volume of O_2 for each g Hb
    _____ Total arterial oxygen content
    _____ Total venous oxygen content
    _____ Arterial-venous oxygen content difference
    _____ Oxygen extraction ratio
    _____ Dissolved arterial oxygen content
    _____ Dissolved venous oxygen content

    A. 20 ml/dl
    B. 5 ml/dl
    C. 0.25
    D. 0.3 ml/dl
    E. 15 ml/dl
    F. 1.34 ml
    G. 0.12 ml/dl

20. If hemoglobin = 12 g/dl, SaO_2 = 95%, and PaO_2 = 95 mm Hg, calculate the CaO_2.

21. If hemoglobin = 14 g/dl, SaO_2 = 90%, PaO_2 = 65 mm Hg, $S\bar{v}O_2$ = 68%, and $P\bar{v}O_2$ = 40 mm Hg, calculate the oxygen extraction ratio.

III. Oxygen Transport to the Tissues

22. The only way the body normally increases oxygen delivery to the tissues is by:
    A. Increasing cardiac output
    B. Increasing PO_2
    C. Increasing SaO_2
    D. Increasing CaO_2

23. Normal resting oxygen extraction by the tissues:
    A. Is about 10% of oxygen delivered to the tissues
    B. Is 250 ml/min
    C. Returns 500 ml oxygen/min to venous circulation
    D. Returns 50% of delivered oxygen to venous circulation

IV. Cyanosis

24. Cyanosis is usually visible when:
    A. At least 5 g/dl of capillary hemoglobin is desaturated
    B. Venous hemoglobin is 25% desaturated
    C. Hemoglobin concentration is less than 10 g/dl
    D. Average capillary hemoglobin concentration is 5% desaturated

25. Central cyanosis differs from peripheral cyanosis because:
    A. Central cyanosis is visible only on the lips and membranes of the mouth
    B. Central cyanosis is caused by excessively low SaO_2
    C. Peripheral cyanosis is caused by inadequate blood oxygenation in the lung
    D. Peripheral cyanosis is usually visible in any capillary bed

V. Hemoglobin Abnormalities

26. Methemoglobin:
    A. Has low affinity for oxygen compared to normal hemoglobin
    B. Contains oxidized iron
    C. Crystallizes when deoxygenated
    D. Is normally present in the newborn

27. Sickle cell hemoglobin:
    A. Binds irreversibly with oxygen
    B. Contains oxidized iron
    C. Crystallizes when deoxygenated
    D. Is normally present in the newborn

▶ Putting It All Together

1. A patient with a structural heart defect has chronic polycythemia and a hemoglobin concentration of 22 g/dl. How much deoxyhemoglobin must be present for cyanosis to occur?

2. Clinicians sometimes omit part of the oxygen content formula and use only "[Hb] × 1.34 ml O_2/g Hb × SO_2." How can this shortened formula be a useful reflection of oxygen content?

3. A patient with a hemoglobin concentration of 8.0 has an SaO_2 of 94%. Which of the following improves the patient's oxygen delivery more: increasing the SaO_2 to 100% with supplemental oxygen or transfusing blood to increase the hemoglobin concentration to 10 g/dl?

4. Comment on the way oxygen content is affected when SaO_2 is increased from 90% to 99% (without changing hemoglobin concentration) versus increasing hemoglobin concentration from 10 g/dl to 11 g/dl (without changing SaO_2).

5. A patient suffering from prolonged smoke inhalation has an SpO_2 (measured by portable pulse oximeter) of 100% and an SaO_2 (measured by CO oximeter) of 80%. The patient appears "flushed" with rosy skin color. Explain the difference between the two oxygen saturation values and how this difference may be associated with the patient's skin color.

6. An adequately hydrated patient has a hemoglobin concentration of 15, an SaO_2 of 97%, a PaO_2 of 98 mm Hg, a cardiac output of 2.8 L/min, and a venous oxygen content of 9.5 ml/dl. The low venous oxygen content is the result of:
    A. Abnormal hemoglobin
    B. Low arterial oxygen content
    C. Hypovolemia
    D. Low cardiac output

7. During septicemia (blood infection), tissue oxygen demands may increase dramatically. The oxyhemoglobin curve shift most advantageous in this situation is (right, left). In this case, which factors are present to cause a shift?

▶ Cases to Consider

1. As the RCP working in a trauma care unit, you are asked to obtain an arterial blood sample from a motor vehicle accident victim to evaluate the patient's ventilation and oxygenation. The patient sustained multiple injuries that have resulted in significant blood loss (Hb = 6.0); this is treated with a blood transfusion. On supplemental oxygen, the patient's spontaneous breathing frequency and tidal volumes appear to be below normal, secondary to the ventilation-depressive effects of analgesic medication. The arterial blood gas analysis before the blood transfusion reveals: PaO_2 = 75, SaO_2 = 88%, below normal pH, and above normal $PaCO_2$. While reporting the results of the arterial blood gas analysis to the attending physician, you comment that the oxyhemoglobin curve in this patient is shifted, because of hypoventilation. State which direction the curve shifted, the reason for the shift, and what action may help correct the abnormal blood gas values.

2. You have provided the patient in the case above with nasal positive airway pressure to correct hypoventilation. Banked blood has been transfused to correct the patient's hypovolemia and abnormally low hemoglobin (Hb after transfusion is 12.0). One hour after the initial arterial blood analysis was performed, you draw another sample. The results of this sample are: PO_2 = 70; SaO_2 = 98%; PCO_2 and pH are now within normal limits. Comment on the position of the oxyhemoglobin curve, the reason for its position, and why the hemoglobin oxygen content has changed from 1 hour ago.

3. A post-operative cardiac surgery patient has just arrived to the coronary care unit and you are the RCP in attendance. The patient's body temperature on arrival to the unit is 35° C, which is common after this type of surgery. After 30 minutes of mechanical ventilation, you draw an arterial blood gas sample. The results are: PaO_2 = 65, SaO_2 = 98%, $PaCO_2$ = 40, pH = 7.4, and Hb = 13. The cardiac output measurement you performed shortly before the arterial blood gas analysis showed an output of 4.8 L/min. The attending physician, noting the cardiac output measurement and the apparent discrepancy between the PaO_2 and SaO_2 of the blood gas sample, asks you if the patient's tissue oxygen delivery is adequate for tissue oxygen consumption. While answering, you request that the patient be warmed to 37° C and that a venous blood sample be drawn. Defend your requests.

4. You draw a mixed venous blood sample from the Swan-Ganz catheter's distal port in the patient in the case above. The results of the analyzed sample are: $P\bar{v}O_2$ = 38 mm Hg, $S\bar{v}O_2$ = 60%, and Hb = 13 g/dl. Calculate the tissue oxygen consumption rate and oxygen extraction ratio.

Chapter 9

Carbon Dioxide Equilibrium and Transport

▷ Points to Remember

- Blood carbon dioxide is produced by tissue metabolism.
- P_ACO_2 and $PaCO_2$ concentrations are maintained at about 40 mm Hg by alveolar CO_2 elimination; the CO_2 elimination rate normally equals CO_2 production.
- CO_2 in the blood forms H_2CO_3, which dissociates into H^+ and HCO_3^- ions.
- $PaCO_2$ reflects blood volatile acid content and alveolar ventilation adequacy.
- Hypoventilation (high P_ACO_2) and hyperventilation (low P_ACO_2) are abnormal CO_2 equilibrium states in which CO_2 production and elimination rates are equal.
- Ventilatory work may be so high in severe obstructive airways disease that the body tolerates persistent hypoventilation and acidemia to conserve energy.
- CO_2 in the blood is carried in three major forms: as dissolved CO_2, as bicarbonate ions, and as carbamino compounds.
- Most blood CO_2 is carried as HCO_3^- ions in the plasma; however, HCO_3^- is mainly generated in the red blood cells.
- As oxygen dissociates from hemoglobin, its affinity for CO_2 is increased at the tissue level (Haldane effect). As CO_2 enters the blood, hemoglobin affinity for oxygen decreases (Bohr effect).

▷ The Basics

I. Carbon Dioxide, Carbonic Acid, and Hydrogen Ion Equilibrium

1. Average tissue PCO_2 is approximately:
   A. 100 mm Hg
   B. 46 mm Hg
   C. 40 mm Hg
   D. 60 mm Hg

2. The concentration of CO_2 in the blood leaving systemic capillaries is:
   A. Greater than the tissue CO_2 concentration
   B. Less than the CO_2 concentration in blood leaving the pulmonary capillary bed
   C. Less than the tissue CO_2 concentration
   D. Greater than the average alveolar CO_2

3. Complete the following CO_2 hydration equation:

   $$H_2O + CO_2 \longrightarrow \longrightarrow$$

4. At equilibrium in plasma, the CO_2 hydration equation:
   A. Is shifted to the left
   B. Has equal substance concentrations on both sides
   C. Is shifted to the right
   D. Has greater left-directed reaction rates

5. Complete the figure below by filling in the appropriate normal resting values for CO_2 production, CO_2 elimination, alveolar CO_2, and plasma $PaCO_2$.

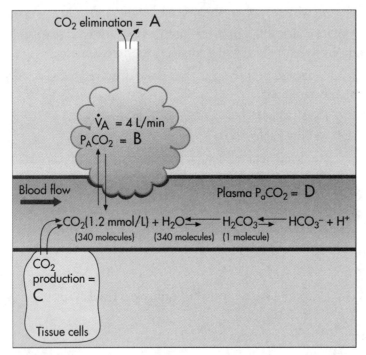

6. From the following events, select only those that occur during hypoventilation, and number them sequentially as they occur over time.
   _____ Alveolar PCO_2 decreases.
   _____ Plasma PCO_2 increases.
   _____ Alveolar PCO_2 increases.
   _____ Dissolved CO_2 increases.
   _____ H_2CO_3 concentration increases.
   _____ H_2CO_3 concentration decreases.

7. Label the two illustrations below as either hypoventilation or hyperventilation; state the direction of shift in the CO_2 hydration reaction; and identify the CO_2 production/elimination ratio at the new equilibrium point.

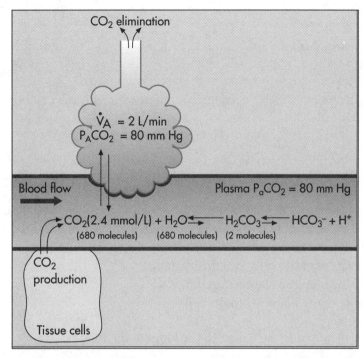

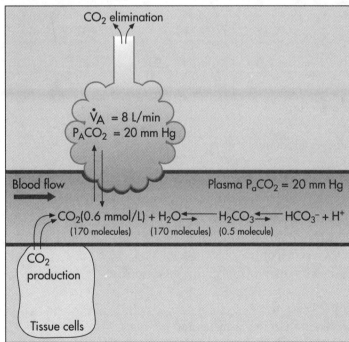

8. All of the following are consistent with an alkalemic state secondary to increased ventilation *except*:
   A. $P_ACO_2 < 40$ mm Hg
   B. $PaCO_2 < 40$ mm Hg
   C. Elevated blood carbonic acid
   D. Low H^+ ion concentration

II. How Blood Carries Carbon Dioxide

9. The major forms of CO_2 carried in the blood include all of the following *except*:
   A. Plasma H_2CO_3
   B. Dissolved CO_2
   C. Carbamino compounds
   D. HCO_3^- ions

10. The most direct determinant of H^+ concentration in the blood is the amount of:
    A. Plasma H_2CO_3
    B. Dissolved CO_2
    C. Carbamino compounds
    D. HCO_3^- ions

11. As a consequence of hemoglobin buffering hydrogen ions, HCO_3^- ions diffuse from erythrocytes into plasma, creating an electrical imbalance that is subsequently neutralized by:
    A. Na^+ ions diffusing out of the cells into the plasma
    B. K^+ ions diffusing out of the cells into the plasma
    C. Cl^- ions diffusing from the plasma into the cells
    D. CO_2 diffusing from the plasma into the cells

12. Most CO_2 is transported from the tissues to the lungs in the form of:
    A. Plasma H_2CO_3
    B. Dissolved CO_2
    C. Carbamino compounds
    D. Plasma HCO_3^- ions

13. Some CO_2 reacts with NH_2 groups of plasma proteins to form:
    A. Carbamino-hemoglobin
    B. Plasma H_2CO_3
    C. Plasma carbamino compounds
    D. Plasma HCO_3^- ions

14. Which is true of oxygen combining with heme groups on the hemoglobin molecule?
    A. Hemoglobin affinity for CO_2 is enhanced.
    B. This occurs more readily when carbamino compounds are bound to hemoglobin.
    C. This decreases CO_2 transport capacity of the blood.
    D. This enhances the formation of carbamino-hemoglobin.

15. Carbon dioxide concentration is:
    A. Lower in whole blood than in plasma alone
    B. Greater in the red blood cells than in plasma
    C. Equivalent in red blood cells and plasma
    D. Greater in whole blood than in plasma alone

▷ Putting It All Together

1. If tissue metabolism increases and alveolar ventilation remains normal, CO_2 (increases, decreases), H^+ ion concentration (increases, decreases), and pH (increases, decreases).

2. Indicate if the following statements about hyperventilation are true (T) or false (F).
   _____ Increased alveolar carbon dioxide partial pressure
   _____ Decreased plasma carbon dioxide partial pressure
   _____ Decreased carbonic acid
   _____ Increased hydrogen ion concentration
   _____ Right-shifted hydration reaction
   _____ Left-shifted hydration equilibrium point
   _____ Normal carbon dioxide tissue production/alveolar elimination ratio

3. An arterial blood gas analysis of a patient breathing room air provides these results: PO_2 = 55 mm Hg and PCO_2 = 34 mm Hg. Without other clinical data, this information suggests that the patient:
   A. Is hypoxemic secondary to hypoventilation
   B. Has chronic obstructive airways disease with alveolar CO_2 retention
   C. Is hyperventilating secondary to hypoxemia
   D. Has a blood carbonic acid level above normal

4. In anemic patients, the red blood cell H^+ ion buffering capacity is (increased, decreased).

▷ Cases to Consider

1. Mechanical ventilation has just begun for a cardiac arrest patient who was successfully resuscitated 10 minutes ago. An arterial blood gas analysis reveals a PO_2 of 110 mm Hg, a PCO_2 of 38 mm Hg, and a pH of 7.25. A laboratory blood sample reveals very high lactic acid levels following the resuscitative efforts. The attending physician requests your input to appropriately change the patient's mechanical ventilation. How can changing the patient's ventilation improve the clinical picture and why?

2. Appropriate changes have been made to the mechanical ventilator of the patient in the case above. Two hours after increasing the patient's breathing frequency, a follow-up arterial blood gas analysis reveals a PO_2 of 115 mm Hg, a PCO_2 of 29 mm Hg, and a pH of 7.5. Since the physician left instructions to "titrate breathing frequency according to blood gas results," is there a change indicated and, if so, what change should be made?

Chapter 10
Acid-Base Regulation

▷ Points To Remember

- Hydrogen ions are produced continuously by aerobic metabolism.
- Blood buffers are classified as bicarbonate (open) or nonbicarbonate (closed) systems.
- Hemoglobin is the major buffer of the closed nonbicarbonate blood buffer system
- Plasma HCO_3^- buffers more H^+ ions than any other blood buffer.
- The open bicarbonate buffer system buffers H^+ more effectively than the closed nonbicarbonate buffer system because in the open system, ventilation continually removes CO_2, allowing continual buffering of H^+ by HCO_3^-.
- In the closed nonbicarbonate system, H^+ ion buffering slows or stops as the concentrations of reactants and products reach equilibrium.
- Ventilation is intimately involved in acid-base regulation because it directly affects blood CO_2 levels.
- The kidneys participate in maintaining a constant pH by excreting H^+ or by conserving HCO_3^-.
- According to the Henderson-Hasselbalch equation, the relationship between $[HCO_3^-]$ and dissolved CO_2 determines the pH; a 20:1 $[HCO_3^-]$ to dissolved CO_2 ratio always produces a pH of 7.40 in blood plasma.
- The lungs control the dissolved CO_2 in the plasma and the kidneys control plasma $[HCO_3^-]$.
- "Metabolic" (or nonrespiratory) acid-base disturbances occur when $[HCO_3^-]$ changes are the main reason for changes in pH.
- Respiratory acid-base imbalances occur when $PaCO_2$ changes are the main reason for changes in pH.
- An imbalance in either the metabolic or respiratory acid-base components elicits a compensatory response by the other component so that normal pH is restored.
- The CO_2 hydration reaction causes $[HCO_3^-]$ to increase slightly when PCO_2 increases (an increase separate from that due to renal HCO_3^- retention).

▸ The Basics

I. Concepts of Acids, Bases, and pH

1. The following is true of protein molecules:
   A. They are positively charged (polycations).
   B. They maintain a constant shape as they combine with H^+ ions.
   C. They are structural components of intracellular enzymes.
   D. They do not combine readily with H^+ ions.

2. The following is true of the hydrogen ion:
   A. It is a hydrogen atom with one electron.
   B. It exists as H_3O^+ in aqueous fluids.
   C. It reacts with positively charged regions of protein molecules.
   D. It exists as a simple proton in aqueous body fluids.

3. Alkalosis refers to:
   A. An accumulation of H^+ in body fluids
   B. Body fluids with a subnormal pH
   C. Higher than normal amounts of proton acceptors in body fluids
   D. Reduced concentrations of base in body fluids

4. The following is true of a strong acid:
   A. It ionizes only slightly in an aqueous solution.
   B. It has a pH greater than 7.0.
   C. It has a low dissociation velocity according to the law of mass action.
   D. It has a large equilibrium constant.

5. The following is true of pH:
   A. It is the exponent of $[H^+]$.
   B. It is the negative logarithm of $[H^+]$.
   C. It decreases as $[H^+]$ decreases.
   D. It is 7.4 for a chemically neutral solution.

6. When pH changes in the normal physiologic range by 0.01, $[H^+]$ changes by about:
   A. 0.1 nM/L
   B. 1 nM/L
   C. 10 nM/L
   D. 100 nM/L

II. Body Buffer Systems

7. Aerobic metabolism normally generates 13,000 mM of CO_2 daily. This, in turn, produces a daily H^+ quantity of:
   A. 130 mM
   B. 1,300 mM
   C. 13,000 mM
   D. 130,000 mM

8. All of the following are fixed acids *except*:
   A. Sulfuric acid
   B. Lactic acid
   C. Phosphoric acid
   D. Carbonic acid

9. The respiratory system compensates for fixed acid accumulation by:
   A. Eliminating CO_2 and shifting the hydration reaction to the left
   B. Eliminating fixed acids directly through increased ventilation
   C. Increasing buffer concentration by increasing CO_2 elimination
   D. Retaining H_2CO_3 and shifting the hydration reaction to the right

10. The closed buffer system includes phosphates and:
    A. Hemoglobin
    B. H_2CO_3
    C. Plasma HCO_3^-
    D. Erythrocyte HCO_3^-

11. When a given quantity of H+ is added to a bicarbonate buffer solution, the pH change:
    A. Is greatest when the solution contains 50% HCO_3^- and 50% dissolved CO_2
    B. Is greatest if the solution's pH is similar to the solution's pK
    C. Is smallest when added to a solution containing 50% CO_2 and 50% HCO_3^-
    D. Is greatest when the solution's pH is equal to 6.1

12. If all other variables remain constant in the Henderson-Hasselbalch equation, an increase in dissolved CO_2 will (increase, decrease) pH.

13. If all other variables remain constant in the Henderson-Hasselbalch equation, an increase in $[HCO_3^-]$ will (increase, decrease) blood alkalinity.

14. Which of the following is true of the bicarbonate buffering system?
    A. It effectively buffers volatile acids.
    B. It is normally unable to buffer lactic acid.
    C. It buffers carbonic acid during hypoventilation.
    D. It relies on CO_2 production to replenish bicarbonate buffer stores.

15. H+ cannot be buffered after equilibrium is reached between buffers and their products in the (bicarbonate, nonbicarbonate) system.

16. Which of the following is true of HCO_3^- buffers?
    A. They are normally used up when buffering fixed acids.
    B. They are regenerated, in part, by hemoglobin's buffering of H^+.
    C. They are replenished by CO_2's reaction with H_2CO_3.
    D. They cannot be used when equilibrium between buffers and buffer products is reached.

III. Henderson-Hasselbalch Equation

17. The Henderson-Hasselbalch equation substitutes which term for [H_2CO_3]?
    A. [H^+]
    B. Dissolved CO_2 (mmol/L)
    C. pK
    D. $PaCO_2$ (mm Hg)

18. If a patient's arterial blood gas has a HCO_3^- of 24 mEq/L and a $PaCO_2$ of 45 mm Hg, calculate the blood pH.

19. If the pH = 7.29 and the $PaCO_2$ = 30 mm Hg, calculate the HCO_3^-.

20. If the pH = 7.52 and the [HCO_3^-] = 24, calculate the $PaCO_2$.

21. The HCO_3^- value obtained from an analyzed arterial blood sample is:
    A. Measured; and $PaCO_2$ and pH are computed
    B. Computed, as is pH
    C. Computed; and $PaCO_2$ and pH are measured
    D. Measured, as is $PaCO_2$

IV. Acid Excretion

22. Lungs eliminate the CO_2 produced by:
    A. The open buffer system only
    B. Fixed acids only
    C. Volatile and fixed acids
    D. Volatile acids only

23. When blood PCO_2 is high, the kidneys excrete:
    A. Greater amounts of H^+ and smaller amounts of HCO_3^-
    B. Smaller amounts of H^+ and greater amounts of HCO_3^-
    C. Greater amounts of both H^+ and HCO_3^-
    D. Smaller amounts of both H^+ and HCO_3^-

V. Acid-Base Disturbances

24. Blood pH equals 7.40 if:
    A. HCO_3^- = 20 and $PaCO_2$ = 36
    B. HCO_3^- = 26 and $PaCO_2$ = 38
    C. HCO_3^- = 30 and $PaCO_2$ = 46
    D. HCO_3^- = 30 and $PaCO_2$ = 50

25. Respiratory alkalosis is caused by:
    A. Decreased HCO_3^- excretion
    B. Increased CO_2 excretion
    C. Hypoventilation
    D. [HCO_3^-] : ($PaCO_2$ x 0.03) ratio less than 20 : 1

26. Metabolic acid-base disturbances are caused primarily by:
    A. Gains or losses in plasma HCO_3^- only
    B. Changes in the denominator of the Henderson-Hasselbalch equation
    C. Increases or decreases in dissolved CO_2
    D. Gains or losses of fixed acids or HCO_3^-

27. Causes of metabolic alkalosis include all of the following *except:*
    A. Sodium bicarbonate ingestion
    B. Excessive vomiting
    C. Diarrhea
    D. Loss of fixed acids

28. Complete the following table, indicating in each disorder whether HCO_3^- and PCO_2 remain unchanged, increase, or decrease. Supply the same information for the compensatory response to each disorder.

Acid-Base Disorder	Primary Defect	Compensatory Response
Respiratory acidosis		
Respiratory alkalosis		
Metabolic acidosis		
Metabolic alkalosis		

▶ Putting It All Together

1. A patient who has been non-compliant with her insulin therapy experiences an episode of ketoacidosis (ketones are acids produced by fat metabolism). Her symptoms include increased breathing frequency and large tidal volumes. Why?

2. Why does a patient with arterial blood gas results such as those provided in question 19 in "The Basics" section have an abnormally low $PaCO_2$ of 30 mm Hg?

3. Why does the patient in question 20 in "The Basics" section have an abnormally low $PaCO_2$ of approximately 30 mm Hg?

4. Individuals experiencing acute, severe metabolic acidosis often require some form of ventilatory support before the primary cause of their acidosis is corrected. Why is this so, and when should ventilatory support be initiated?

5. If the ratio between $[HCO_3^-]$ and dissolved CO_2 is known, it is possible to know whether the acid-base balance tends toward acidosis or alkalosis, even if the pH is not known. Why?

6. Some individuals with COPD have chronically elevated $PaCO_2$, with normal pH. If the $PaCO_2$ = 55 and the pH = 7.4, what is the $[HCO_3^-]$?

7. What will the new pH be for the scenario in question number 6 if the $PaCO_2$ rapidly decreases to 40 mm Hg? Would a patient with the new pH have a normal acid-base balance, be acidotic, or be alkalotic?

▶ Cases to Consider

1. You are the RCP working in a medical intensive care unit when an unresponsive, middle-aged woman is brought in. She has been intubated by the ambulance personnel to protect her airway from inadvertent aspiration of gastric contents. The patient is the pedestrian victim of a motor vehicle accident. While connecting her endotracheal tube to a mechanical ventilator circuit, you notice that the posterior portion of her head is heavily bandaged and that she has an intracranial pressure (ICP) transducer connected to a sensor placed in an opening into her cranium. According to the attending physician, she sustained a "subdural hematoma" (swelling of brain tissue due to broken blood vessels) and her ICP is increased above normal. High ICPs are known to produce permanent brain damage. It is also known that lowering a patient's blood $[H^+]$ reduces ICP. An arterial blood gas is drawn on the current ventilator settings with these results: PaO_2 = 95 mm Hg, $PaCO_2$ = 42 mm Hg, pH = 7.34, HCO_3^- = 22, and SaO_2 = 99%. The attending physician wishes to increase the patient's pH to 7.50 and asks you to assist in attaining this goal. Can you help?

2. The physician in the case above agrees to a target $PaCO_2$ of 29 mm Hg to achieve a pH of 7.50. The patient is heavily sedated and is not initiating spontaneous breaths through the ventilator. The ventilator's set breathing frequency is 10 and the tidal volume is 600 ml. What must the patient's new minute ventilation be to produce a PCO_2 of 29 mm Hg? If breathing frequency remains at 10, what must the tidal volume be for the new minute ventilation?

3. A physician is discussing the current clinical status of an emphysema patient with you. The greatest concern the physician has regarding this otherwise stable patient is that there seems to be an acute loss of HCO_3^-, as represented in today's arterial blood gas results. The results are: PaO_2 = 59 mm Hg, $PaCO_2$ = 50 mm Hg, pH = 7.40, $[HCO_3^-]$ = 22 mEq/L, and SaO_2 = 89%. All of the values in the blood gas report are at the patient's normal baseline except for the low-normal $[HCO_3^-]$, which has been *above* normal in the past (compensatory response to chronically high $PaCO_2$). The physician is considering ordering other laboratory tests to determine the reason for the HCO_3^- depletion. You state that further tests are not necessary, other than possibly redrawing the arterial blood gas. What are the reasons for this statement?

4. If you assume that the $[HCO_3^-]$ in the blood gas report for the patient above is wrong, what do you expect the correct value to be for a $PaCO_2$ of 50 and pH of 7.40?

Chapter 11
Control of Ventilation

▷ Points to Remember

- The respiratory center, consisting of inspiratory and expiratory neurons, is located in the brain's medulla.
- Pontine and medullary chemoreceptor impulses modify the inspiratory and expiratory neuronal output, producing a cyclical ventilatory rhythm.
- Peripheral chemoreceptors, stretch receptors, irritant/pain receptors, and the cerebral cortex modify the rate, depth, and pattern of breathing.
- Muscle spindles produce spinal reflexes that help ventilatory muscles adjust to varying loads.
- Arterial carbon dioxide reacts with water in the the cerebral spinal fluid (CSF), producing chemoreceptor-stimulating H^+ ions that are the primary stimulation for ventilation.
- Arterial hypoxemia becomes the primary ventilatory stimulus in people with chronically high $PaCO_2$s because the kidneys compensate by increasing blood HCO_3^- levels, which normalizes pH.
- The hypoxic drive, mediated by peripheral chemoreceptors, is activated when the PaO_2 is 60 mm Hg or less.
- Supplemental oxygen should be administered cautiously to chronically hypercapnic individuals who are breathing by hypoxic stimulation because oxygen may remove the ventilatory drive.
- Ventilation, oxygen consumption, and carbon dioxide production are so closely matched during exercise that PaO_2, pH, and $PaCO_2$ remain normal during exercise.
- Central nervous system injuries and abnormalities produce specific types of abnormal breathing patterns, altering normal oxygenation and acid-base status.

▶ The Basics

I. The Medullary and Pontine Respiratory Centers

1. Label the diagram of the brain stem with the names of its three main parts and the names of respiratory neuron groups: pneumotaxic center, apneustic center, medulla oblongata, pons, spinal cord, ventral respiratory groups, dorsal respiratory groups, nucleus ambiguus, and nucleus retroambigualis.

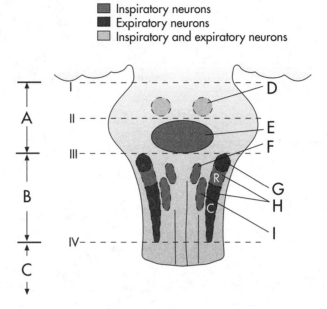

2. Number the following neural inspiratory signal events sequentially as they occur during medullary/pontine-controlled ventilation.
   _____ Progressive contraction of inspiratory muscles
   _____ Inspiratory neuronal activity completely absent; passive lung recoil occurs
   _____ Inspiratory neurons fire briefly, maintaining inspiratory muscle tone
   _____ Firing rate gradually increases from dorsal and ventral inspiratory neurons at the end of the expiratory phase
   _____ Gradual lung expansion
   _____ Inhibitory neurons turn off inspiratory signal

3. Match the respiratory center components on the left with the appropriate descriptions on the right. (Note: One description is used twice.)

   _____ Apneustic center
   _____ Dorsal respiratory group
   _____ Nucleus ambiguus
   _____ Ventral respiratory group
   _____ Pneumotaxic center
   _____ Nucleus retro-ambigualis

   A. Inspiratory neurons innervating laryngeal and pharyngeal muscles
   B. Neurons with expiratory signaling of internal and abdominal muscles and neurons intercostal with DRG-like functions
   C. Neurons located bilaterally in two different nuclei on the medulla
   D. Has neural connections with the pneumotaxic center but its function is poorly understood
   E. Sends impulses to phrenic and external intercostal spinal motor nerves
   F. Limits inspiration and holds apneustic signals in check

II. Reflex Control of Breathing

4. Which of the following is true of the Hering-Breuer reflex?
   A. It is stimulated mainly during expiration.
   B. It is generated by stimulation of airway smooth muscle stretch receptors.
   C. It switches on the inspiratory ramp signal.
   D. It is an important control mechanism in quiet breathing.

5. Which of the following is true of the interaction between low lung compliance and neuronal control of respiration?
   A. It decreases airway distending pressure, decreasing stretch receptor stimulation.
   B. It results in stretch receptor stimulation, increasing the inspiratory phase.
   C. It may increase breathing frequency because stretch receptor stimulation shortens the inspiratory phase.
   D. It increases respiratory rate because stretch receptors shorten the expiratory phase.

6. All of the following are true about Head's reflex *except*:
   A. The reflex receptors are called rapidly adapting receptors.
   B. Head's reflex helps maintain large tidal volumes during exercise.
   C. Head's reflex causes responses similar to Hering-Breuer reflex responses.
   D. The reflex is involved in periodic deep sighs during quiet breathing.

7. Match the terms on the left with the appropriate descriptions on the right.

   _____ Rapidly adapting irritant receptors
   _____ Vagovagal reflexes
   _____ Juxtacapillary receptors
   _____ Peripheral proprioceptors
   _____ Deflation reflex
   _____ Hering-Breuer reflex
   _____ Slowly adapting receptors

   A. C-fibers near pulmonary capillaries that cause rapid, shallow breathing
   B. Stretch receptors that generate the Hering-Breuer reflex
   C. Located in large airway epithelium
   D. Only activated at large volumes in adults
   E. Responsible for hyperpnea with pneumothorax
   F. Located in muscles, tendons, and joints
   G. Reflexes with both sensory and motor vagal components

8. Painful stimuli and limb movement produce ventilation in patients with respiratory depression because of stimulatory signals sent by:
   A. Proprioceptors
   B. Irritant receptors
   C. Rapidly adapting receptors
   D. Chemoreceptors

9. A reflex arc helps the diaphragm and intercostal muscles adjust to increased work of breathing. Number the following reflex arc events in the order of occurrence.
   _____ Main extrafusal and intrafusal fibers contract in parallel.
   _____ Stretch-sensitive spindle is unloaded and its impulses cease.
   _____ Main extrafusal muscle contracts, shortening nearby intrafusal muscle fibers.
   _____ Spinal cord sends impulses back to the main extrafusal muscle.
   _____ The spindle sensing element stretches and sends impulses over afferent nerves to the spinal cord.

III. Chemical Control Of Ventilation

10. Central and peripheral chemoreceptors stimulate ventilation because of all of the following *except*:
    A. Hypercapnia
    B. Hypoxia
    C. Alkalemia
    D. Acidemia

11. Peripheral chemoreceptors respond to:
    A. Hypoxia and hydrogen ions
    B. Arterial hydrogen ions and carbon dioxide
    C. Arterial carbon dioxide and hypoxia
    D. Arterial carbon dioxide, hypoxia, and hydrogen ions

12. Medullary (central) chemoreceptors respond to:
    A. Hypoxia and hydrogen ions
    B. Hydrogen ions generated by arterial carbon dioxide
    C. Arterial carbon dioxide and hypoxia
    D. Arterial carbon dioxide, hypoxia, and hydrogen ions

13. Central chemoreceptors are in direct contact with:
    A. Cerebrospinal fluid (CSF)
    B. Arterial blood
    C. The blood-brain barrier
    D. H+ diffusing from arterial blood

14. Minute-to-minute central chemoreceptor control of ventilation is the *direct* result of changes in _____ and the *indirect* result of changes in _____.

15. Arterial carbon dioxide concentration stimulates central chemoreceptors through all of the following mechanisms *except*:
    A. Arterial H+ ion diffusion across the blood-brain barrier
    B. Formation of HCO_3^- in the CSF
    C. Arterial CO_2 diffusion across the blood-brain barrier
    D. Formation of carbonic acid in the CSF

16. The carotid bodies increase neural firing rates in response to decreased arterial:
    A. PO_2
    B. O_2 content
    C. PCO_2
    D. [H⁺]

17. Ventilatory increases initiated by stimulation of the carotid bodies are held in check by:
    A. Decreased PO_2
    B. Decreased O_2 content
    C. Increased PCO_2
    D. Increased pH

18. The following events establish hypoxia-driven ventilation in chronic hypercapnia. Number the events in order of occurrence.
    _____ Plasma $[HCO_3^-]$ increases.
    _____ P_ACO_2 is chronically high.
    _____ Arterial PCO_2 and [H⁺] is high.
    _____ Hypercapnic ventilatory drive is removed.
    _____ CSF pH returns to normal.
    _____ HCO_3^- is retained by the kidneys.
    _____ Hypoxemia is the primary ventilatory drive.
    _____ CSF PCO_2 is high.
    _____ Arterial pH returns to normal.
    _____ CSF $[HCO_3^-]$ increases.

IV. Ventilatory Response to Exercise

19. Carbon dioxide production and oxygen consumption increase during exercise. Arterial blood gases during exercise normally show:
    A. Increased PCO_2
    B. Increased PCO_2 and pH
    C. Decreased PO_2
    D. Normal pH

20. Theories about the mechanisms normally responsible for increasing ventilation during exercise include all of the following *except*:
    A. The cerebral motor cortex sends excitatory impulses to exercising muscles and medullary centers.
    B. Abnormal arterial carbon dioxide and oxygen gases stimulate central chemoreceptors, increasing ventilation.
    C. Increased ventilation at the onset of exercise is a learned response.
    D. Exercising limbs stimulate proprioceptors, sending excitatory impulses to medullary centers.

V. Abnormal Breathing Patterns

21. What is the main reason congestive heart failure may cause a Cheyne-Stokes breathing pattern?
    A. Low blood flow causes brain PCO_2 to lag behind lung PCO_2.
    B. This condition increases intracranial pressure, damaging the brain.
    C. This condition may cause pulmonary edema, stimulating the J-receptors.
    D. Low blood flow inadequately oxygenates the brain, adversely affecting central chemoreceptors.

22. Hypoventilation accompanying closed head injuries and central nervous system damage may result in further brain damage because:
    A. Decreased $PaCO_2$ constricts cerebral vessels.
    B. Increased $PaCO_2$ lowers intracranial pressure.
    C. Increased blood $[H^+]$ increases cerebral blood flow.
    D. Decreased blood $[H^+]$ lowers intracranial pressure.

▷ Putting It All Together

1. Patients receiving central nervous system-depressing analgesic medications (such as morphine) may exhibit an acute increase in $PaCO_2$ similar to acute $PaCO_2$ increases in chronically hypercapnic patients with chronic obstructive pulmonary disease who are given high concentrations of oxygen. In what way are these situations similar? In what way do they differ?

2. How do arterial blood gas values during exercise compare to normal resting values and why does this relationship exist?

3. On the illustration of the medulla, circle the blood and CSF chemicals with concentrations that are out of normal range in stable, chronically hypercapnic patients. Characterize the blood and CSF pH in this instance.

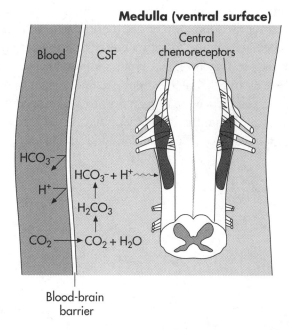

4. Consider the person with a traumatic head injury and increased intracranial pressures (ICP). State the primary reason for the increased ICP, why the increased ICP causes further brain damage, and the mechanism by which mechanical hyperventilation reduces ICP.

5. In what way is acid-base compensation in chronic hypercapnia similar to what happens to the ICP-reducing effects of mechanical hyperventilation after about 48 hours?

▶ Cases to Consider

1. A patient with chronic obstructive pulmonary disease with chronic hypercapnia is on the orthopedic surgical unit after total hip replacement surgery. As the respiratory care practitioner for the unit, you are providing the patient's maintenance regimen of inhaled bronchodilators and steroids. Because of the patient's pulmonary history, a preoperative arterial blood gas sample was drawn and analyzed while the patient breathed a supplemental oxygen flow of 1 L/min. Blood gas results at that time were: PO_2 = 58 mm Hg, PCO_2 = 50 mm Hg, SaO_2 = 89, pH = 7.36, and HCO_3^- = 27.3 mEq/L. Postoperatively the patient is receiving self-administered analgesics (pain relievers) for pain and is on supplemental oxygen at 1 L/min. On the first postoperative day, the patient's surgeon analyzes the electrolytes and notices that total CO_2 (dissolved CO_2 and CO_2 carried as HCO_3^-) is above normal. The patient is alert and breathing at his normal rate of 20 breaths per minute. The surgeon requests that a blood gas be drawn to evaluate this individual's ventilatory status. The arterial blood gas results on 1 L/min oxygen are: PO_2 = 59, PCO_2 = 51 mm Hg, SaO_2 = 89, pH = 7.35, and HCO_3^- = 27 mEq/L. The surgeon reviews the blood gas results and, because the $PaCO_2$ is above normal, is concerned that the patient may be using excessive amounts of pain medication, which is depressing the drive to breathe. What is your assessment of the patient's ventilatory status?

2. The patient in the case above is now in his fourth postoperative day and is using only small amounts of pain medications. Physical therapists have been walking with the patient since the second postoperative day. Your are paged by one of the physical therapists to evaluate the patient in his room. When you enter the room, you notice that the patient is lethargic and arouses only briefly when his name is spoken loudly. You also observe that the patient's nasal oxygen cannula is still in place and that oxygen flow is set at 2 L/min. A portable pulse oximeter probe attached to the patient's finger reveals an SpO_2 of 95% (pulse oximeter margin of error is ±3%) with a breathing frequency of 12. You reduce the oxygen flow to 1 L/min, continue to monitor the patient's ventilatory status, and state that the patient may be ready to ambulate in 30 minutes, pending a follow-up SpO_2 check. Justify your actions and statement.

Chapter 12
Ventilation-Perfusion Relationships and Arterial Blood Gases

▷ Points to Remember

- *Shunt* refers to alveoli with blood flow but no ventilation; *deadspace* refers to alveoli with ventilation but no blood flow.
- The distribution of individual alveolar $\dot{V}_A/\dot{Q}_C$ ratios determines the overall ratio between air and blood flow in the lung.
- Low $\dot{V}_A/\dot{Q}_C$ ratios (< 1.0) are associated wtih impaired blood flow and produce deadspace-like conditions.
- Low $\dot{V}_A/\dot{Q}_C$ ratios always cause hypoxemia but not always hypercapnia.
- High $\dot{V}_A/\dot{Q}_C$ ratios (> 1.0) are associated with impaired blood flow and produce deadspacelike conditions.
- High $\dot{V}_A/\dot{Q}_C$ ratios cause inefficient CO_2 elimination.
- $\dot{V}_A/\dot{Q}_C$ mismatch ($\dot{V}_A/\dot{Q}_C$ < 1 but > 0) and shunt ($\dot{V}_A/\dot{Q}_C$ = 0) are low $\dot{V}_A/\dot{Q}_C$ ratio states associated with hypoxemia.
- Hypoxemia produced by $\dot{V}_A/\dot{Q}_C$ mismatch responds well to oxygen therapy.
- The hallmark of shunt is reduced lung compliance with hypoxemia refractory to oxygen therapy.
- The hallmark of deadspace is high $\dot{V}_E$, disproportionate to $PaCO_2$.
- High $\dot{V}/\dot{Q}$ units may compensate for hypercapnia but not hypoxia from low $\dot{V}_A/\dot{Q}_C$ units.
- PaO_2/P_AO_2, $P(A-a)O_2$, and PaO_2/F_IO_2 are indicators for shunt; PaO_2/P_AO_2 is the most stable and useful clinical indicator.
- Only the classic shunt equation $[\dot{Q}_S/\dot{Q}_T = (C_CO_2 - CaO_2)/(C_CO_2 - C\bar{v}O_2)]$ yields an accurate indication of shunt when cardiac output is unstable.

▶ The Basics

I. $\dot{V}_A/\dot{Q}_C$ Ratio as a Determinant of Alveolar PO_2

1. Overall resting $\dot{V}_A/\dot{Q}_C$ ratio of the lung is:
   A. 1.4
   B. 1.2
   C. 1.0
   D. 0.8

2. Alveolar oxygen concentration:
   A. Increases when $\dot{Q}_C$ decreases, relative to $\dot{V}_A$
   B. Decreases when the $\dot{V}_A/\dot{Q}_C$ ratio is greater than normal
   C. Increases when $\dot{V}_A$ decreases relative to $\dot{Q}_C$
   D. Decreases when $\dot{V}_A/\dot{Q}_C$ is greater than 1.0

3. Write in the appropriate alveolar O_2 and CO_2 partial pressures on the illustration below.

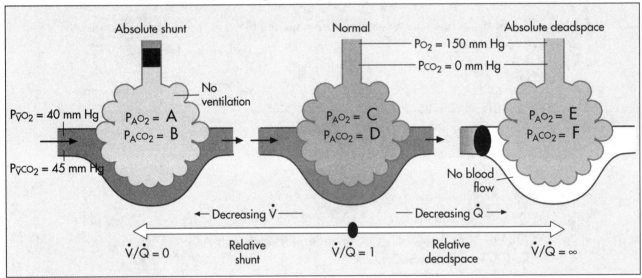

II. The Alveolar Oxygen-Carbon Dioxide Diagram

4. Match the terms on the left with the descriptive terms on the right. (Note: Descriptive terms may be used more than once.)

   _____ Absolute shunt
   _____ Absolute deadspace
   _____ Relative shunt
   _____ Relative deadspace
   _____ Hyperventilation
   _____ Hypoventilation
   _____ Low cardiac output

   A. Shunt-effect (low $\dot{V}_A/\dot{Q}_C$, but > 0)
   B. Deadspace-effect (high $\dot{V}_A/\dot{Q}$, but < infinity)
   C. $\dot{V}_A/\dot{Q}_C$ = infinity
   D. $\dot{V}_A/\dot{Q}_C$ = zero

5. According to the alveolar O_2-CO_2 diagram, P_AO_2 of an absolute shunt alveolus equals:
   A. Mixed venous PO_2
   B. 100 mm Hg
   C. 0 mm Hg
   D. O_2 partial pressure in atmospheric air

6. According to the alveolar O_2-CO_2 diagram, P_ACO_2 of an absolute deadspace alveolus equals:
   A. 40 mm Hg
   B. 0 mm Hg
   C. 45 mm Hg
   D. Mixed venous PCO_2

7. End-capillary blood leaving a normal alveolus that is adequately ventilated with atmospheric air has a PCO_2 equal to:
   A. 40 mm Hg
   B. 0 mm Hg
   C. 45 mm Hg
   D. Mixed venous PCO_2

III. $\dot{V}/\dot{Q}$ Distribution and Imbalances

Use the P_AO_2-P_ACO_2 diagram below to answer questions 8 through 10.

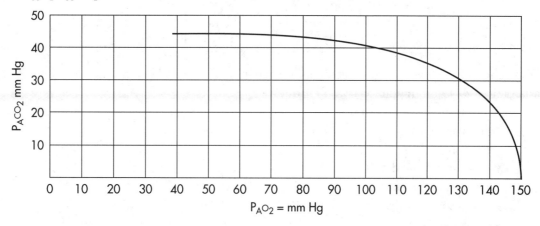

8. Plot points on the P_AO_2-P_ACO_2 curve for absolute shunt, normal $\dot{V}/\dot{Q}$, and absolute deadspace.

9. Beginning with the point on the curve for normal $\dot{V}/\dot{Q}$, use arrows, pointing left or right, and labels to indicate relative deadspace and relative shunt.

10. Indicate the curve segments that represent $\dot{V}/\dot{Q}$ in lung apices and $\dot{V}/\dot{Q}$ in lung bases.

11. Arterial PO_2 is determined by the:
    A. Average of all end-capillary PO_2s
    B. Basal end-capillary O_2 contents
    C. Average of alveolar PO_2
    D. Average of all end-capillary O_2 contents

12. Major V̇/Q̇ imbalance mechanisms causing hypoxemia include all of the following *except*:
    A. Overall hypoventilation
    B. Absolute deadspace
    C. V̇/Q̇ mismatch
    D. Absolute shunt

13. Referring to the figure below, state the primary reason capillary PO_2 is below normal.

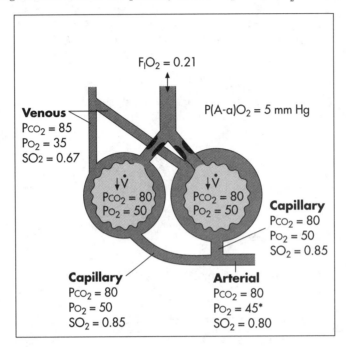

14. For each of the following right-to-left shunt mechanisms, indicate whether it is an example of an anatomic ("A") or intrapulmonary ("P") shunt.
    _____ Atelectasis
    _____ Pulmonary edema
    _____ Pneumonia
    _____ Ventricular septal defect
    _____ Bronchial occlusion
    _____ Adult respiratory distress syndrome
    _____ Airway mucous plug
    _____ Pneumothorax
    _____ Bronchial venous admixture

15. The effect of $\dot{V}_A/\dot{Q}_C$ mismatch on end-capillary blood is:
    A. Low PCO_2 and low PO_2
    B. High PCO_2 and low PO_2
    C. Low PCO_2 and high PO_2
    D. High PCO_2 and high PO_2

16. Which of the following is true regarding $\dot{V}_A/\dot{Q}_C$ mismatches (V̇/Q̇ < 1 but > 0):
    A. It produces deadspacelike conditions and hypoxemia.
    B. It produces high alveolar PCO_2 that results in high PaO_2.
    C. It produces hypoxemia that responds well to oxygen therapy.
    D. The $P(A-a)O_2$ decreases.

17. The PCO_2 in acute $\dot{V}_A/\dot{Q}_C$ mismatch is typically:
    A. Normal to decreased in end-capillary blood from low $\dot{V}_A/\dot{Q}_C$ alveoli
    B. Increased in normal $\dot{V}_A/\dot{Q}_C$ alveoli
    C. Increased in end-capillary blood from normal $\dot{V}_A/\dot{Q}_C$ alveoli
    D. Normal to decreased in arterial blood

18. Normal alveoli in lungs with $\dot{V}_A/\dot{Q}_C$ mismatch and shunt generally develop compensatory:
    A. High $\dot{V}_A/\dot{Q}_C$ ratios
    B. Shuntlike $\dot{V}_A/\dot{Q}_C$ ratios
    C. Decreased minute ventilation
    D. Increased capillary blood flow

19. In the illustration below, blood flow is normal to one lung and absent to the other lung. Indicate what change must occur to return arterial PO_2 and PCO_2 to 100 and 40 mm Hg, respectively, assuming that blood flow distribution remains unchanged.

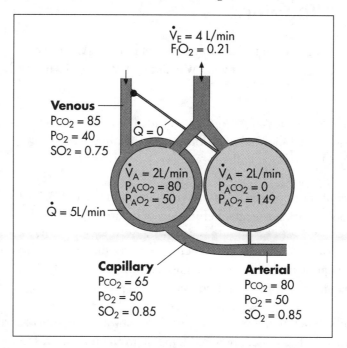

20. Use the Bohr deadspace equation to calculate the percent of minute ventilation used for deadspace ventilation in a patient whose $PaCO_2$ = 40 and P_ECO_2 = 30. Is your answer within normal V_D/V_T limits?

IV. Clinical Measurements of Shunt

21. The only accurate measure of physiologic shunt with unstable cardiac output is the:
    A. A-a gradient
    B. Oxygenation ratio
    C. Classic shunt equation
    D. Percent of P_AO_2 transferred to arterial blood

22. A patient breathing 40% oxygen has a PaO_2 of 67 mm Hg and a $PaCO_2$ of 42 mm Hg in barometric pressure of 760 mm Hg. Calculate the $P(A-a)O_2$. Is shunt present?

23. The lower normal limit for PaO_2/P_AO_2 is:
    A. 1.0
    B. 0.95
    C. 0.8
    D. 0.75

24. If a patient has a PaO_2 of 50 mm Hg and $PaCO_2$ of 35 mm Hg while breathing 25% oxygen and if P_B is 760 mm Hg, what is the F_IO_2 required to increase the PaO_2 to 70 mm Hg?

25. Using the classic shunt equation, calculate the percent shunt for a patient with the following arterial and venous blood gas values: PaO_2 = 65 mm Hg, $PaCO_2$ = 38 mm Hg, SaO_2 = 91%, $P\bar{v}O_2$ = 30 mm Hg, $S\bar{v}O_2$ = 58%, Hb = 14 g/dl, F_IO_2 = 0.21, P_B = 760 mm Hg. State whether the percent shunt is abnormal.

▶ Putting It All Together

1. The $\dot{V}_A/\dot{Q}_C$ ratio changed from normal in the normal lung in Question 19 above, returning the arterial PO_2 and PCO_2 to normal. In what way did it change, and what is the new V_A/Q_C condition called?

2. In Question 19 above, the unperfused lung is exposed to the same increase in ventilation as the normal lung. Answer the following questions about the unperfused lung:
    A. What is its $\dot{V}_A/\dot{Q}_C$ condition called?
    B. What is its $\dot{V}_A/\dot{Q}_C$ ratio?
    C. What direct contribution does its gas make to arterial PO_2 and PCO_2?
    D. In what way does its presence affect efficiency of breathing? Why?

3. A patient with impaired diaphragm movement (such as a diaphragm "flattened" from hyperinflated lungs or a diaphragm that has been paralyzed by a spinal cord injury) is at increased risk for developing hypoxemia when relative deadspace is also present. Why?

4. A patient with lobar pneumonia has some alveoli filled with infectious debris, changing the $\dot{V}_A/\dot{Q}_C$ from normal. This produces regional hypoxia in the lung. In response to regional hypoxemia, pulmonary vasoconstriction occurs in the affected lung area, causing another change in the $\dot{V}_A/\dot{Q}_C$. Is the $\dot{V}_A/\dot{Q}_C$ change caused by alveolar filling relative shunt or relative deadspace? Why does vasoconstriction cause the $\dot{V}_A/\dot{Q}_C$ to change again, and in what way does it change?

5. Positive end-expiratory pressure (PEEP) is often used to improve oxygenation in patients with reduced lung compliance and alveolar collapse. Excessively high PEEP levels, however, may reduce cardiac output. What type of $\dot{V}_A/\dot{Q}_C$ ratio is present before PEEP is initiated? What happens to the $\dot{V}_A/\dot{Q}_C$ ratio when PEEP reduces the cardiac output?

▶ Cases to Consider

1. You are treating a mildly asthmatic patient, using her maintenance regimen of bronchodilators. She also has a skeletal condition called kyphoscoliosis, a deformity that produces an S-shaped lateral curve in her spine. Because of lung compression and reduced rib cage movement, the patient has restrictive lung function. She is also chronically dependent on 1 L/min oxygen flow by nasal cannula to maintain PaO_2 and SaO_2 within normal limits. While auscultating the patient you notice that she has bilateral inspiratory crackles in both lung bases. A recent spirometry test indicates that her pulmonary function is at her "normal" restrictive level. The attending physician is concerned about the patient's persisting need for supplemental oxygen. She asks if you think that providing more intensive bronchodilator therapy would eliminate the patient's oxygen dependence. How do you respond? What is the reason for oxygen dependence?

2. An epileptic patient has been recently intubated and placed on mechanical ventilation while appropriate medication levels are being determined for control of violent seizures. The patient has no history of pulmonary disease and is expected to be mechanically ventilated for only a short time. Since the patient was intubated in an emergency, 100% oxygen is still being delivered while the first arterial blood gas on mechanical ventilation is drawn. The results are: PaO_2 = 48 mm Hg, $PaCO_2$ = 41 mm Hg, SaO_2 = 80%, and P_B = 760 mm Hg. After obtaining the blood gas results, you quickly perform a physical assessment of the patient and discover that no breath sounds can be auscultated over the left lung. The attending physician requests your interpretation of the source of the patient's hypoxemia and what immediate remedy will correct it. You, as the respiratory care practitioner, reply that carefully withdrawing the endotracheal tube until breath sounds are auscultated on the left side will remedy the problem. What is the mechanism for the patient's hypoxemia? What type of $\dot{V}_A/\dot{Q}_C$ defect is present? What is the $P(A-a)O_2$?

Chapter 13

Clinical Assessment of Acid-Base and Oxygenation Status

▷ Points To Remember

- Systematic evaluation of arterial blood gases includes two distinct steps: acid-base disturbances and oxygenation disturbances.
- Abnormal oxygenation may co-exist with normal acid-base ventilatory status.
- Abnormal ventilatory status breathing room air cannot co-exist with normal oxygenation.
- $PaCO_2$ is a reliable, accurate index of ventilatory status.
- Because $[HCO_3^-]$ is affected by $PaCO_2$ changes, it is not always reliable in indicating metabolic status.
- Standard bicarbonate and expected pH calculations clarify metabolic involvement in acid-base disturbances.
- Anion gap calculations identify gain of acid or loss of base as the cause of metabolic acidosis.
- Assessment of oxygenation involves evaluation of two distinct processes: oxygen transfer efficiency across the lung and evaluation of oxygen transport to the tissues.
- Increased age and altitude decrease the normal range for PaO_2.
- Treatment for oxygenation defects may include supplemental O_2, continuous positive airway pressure (CPAP) and mechanical ventilation with positive end-expiratory pressure (PEEP).
- Prolonged F_IO_2s greater than 50% cause pulmonary and systemic oxygen toxicity.
- PEEP and CPAP are useful in treating hypoxemia caused by intrapulmonary shunting.
- Inverse inspiratory/expiratory ratios with pressure-controlled mechanical ventilation are used in extreme cases of refractory hypoxemia.

▶ The Basics

I. Classifying Acid-Base Disturbances

1. The best indicator of the body's acid-base status in arterial blood gases is:
   A. Partial pressure of carbon dioxide
   B. pH
   C. Bicarbonate ion concentration
   D. Partial pressure of oxygen

2. A pH less than 7.00 will most likely cause:
   A. Coma
   B. Convulsions
   C. Tetany
   D. Neuronal excitability

3. List the four steps to systematic acid-base classification.

4. Complete the following table by writing in the appropriate ranges for each arterial blood gas component.

Component	Classification	Ranges
pH (arterial)	Normal	_____
	Acidemia	_____
	Alkalemia	_____
$PaCO_2$ (mm Hg)	Normal ventilatory status	_____
	Respiratory acidosis (hypoventilation)	_____
	Respiratory alkalosis (hyperventilation)	_____
HCO_3^- (mEq/L)	Normal metabolic status	_____
	Metabolic acidosis	_____
	Metabolic alkalosis	_____

5. If arterial pH is 7.48, $PaCO_2$ is 42 mm Hg, and $[HCO_3^-]$ is 30 mEq/L, then: (acidemia, alkalemia, normal pH) is present, the causative component is ($PaCO_2$, HCO_3^-), the compensating component is ($PaCO_2$, HCO_3^-), and this blood gas is classified as _____.

6. If arterial pH is 7.37, $PaCO_2$ is 48 mm Hg, and $[HCO_3^-]$ is 27 mEq/L, then: (acidemia, alkalemia, normal pH) is present, pH is on the (acidic, alkalotic) side of normal, this represents a (noncompensated, compensated, partially compensated) condition, the compensating component is _____, and this blood gas is classified as _____.

7. If arterial pH is 7.33, PaCO$_2$ is 30 mm Hg, and [HCO$_3^-$] is 15 mEq/L, then: (acidemia, alkalemia, normal pH) is present, the causative component is _____, the compensating component is _____, and the pH is (noncompensated, partially compensated, compensated).

8. If arterial pH is 7.47, PaCO$_2$ is 30 mm Hg, and [HCO$_3^-$] is 21 mEq/L, then: (acidemia, alkalemia, normal pH) is present, the causative component is _____, the compensating component is _____, and the pH is (noncompensated, partially compensated, compensated).

9. A PaCO$_2$ greater than 45 mm Hg is compatible with all of the following *except*:
   A. High carbonic acid levels
   B. Acidemia
   C. Hypoventilation
   D. Hypocapnia

10. An *acute* increase of 10 mm Hg in PaCO$_2$ causes [HCO$_3^-$] to:
    A. Decrease by 1 mEq/L
    B. Decrease by 0.1 mEq/L
    C. Increase by 1 mEq/L
    D. Increase by 0.1 mEq/L

11. The most common cause of hyperventilation (and hypocapnia) in patients with pulmonary disease is:
    A. Hypoxemia
    B. Pneumonia
    C. Bicarbonate depletion
    D. Pulmonary edema

12. The pH imbalance produced by overly aggressive mechanical ventilation is called:
    A. Metabolic acidosis
    B. Metabolic alkalosis
    C. Respiratory alkalosis
    D. Respiratory acidosis

13. For each of the following acid-base conditions, state whether the components are above normal ("high"), below normal ("low"), or within normal limits ("WNL").

	pH	PaCO$_2$	[HCO$_3^-$]
Respiratory			
Acidosis (acute)	_____	_____	_____
Acidosis (chronic)	_____	_____	_____
Alkalosis (acute)	_____	_____	_____
Alkalosis (chronic)	_____	_____	_____
Metabolic			
Acidosis (acute)	_____	_____	_____
Acidosis (chronic)	_____	_____	_____
Alkalosis (acute)	_____	_____	_____
Alkalosis (chronic)	_____	_____	_____
Combined			
Acidosis	_____	_____	_____
Alkalosis	_____	_____	_____

14. Metabolic acidosis is a result of all the following *except:*
    A. Anaerobic metabolism
    B. Severe diarrhea
    C. Excessive diuresis and dehydration
    D. Lactic acid production

15. Metabolic alkalosis is associated with all of the following *except:*
    A. Vomiting
    B. Low salt diet
    C. Gastric suctioning
    D. Ammonium chloride ingestion

16. The normal anion gap range is:
    A. 11 to 24 mEq/L
    B. 9 to 14 mEq/L
    C. 22 to 26 mEq/L
    D. 14 to 25 mEq/L

17. The anion gap is calculated by subtracting the sum of _____ and _____ from _____.

18. An above normal anion gap is caused by an accumulation of:
    A. Fixed acids
    B. Bicarbonate
    C. Chloride ions
    D. Volatile acids

19. An example of nonanion gap metabolic acidosis is:
    A. Lactic acidosis
    B. Salicylate overdose
    C. Diarrhea
    D. Ketoacidosis

20. Number the following events in the order of occurrence as metabolic acidosis develops and is compensated.
    - _5_ Central chemoreceptors are stimulated.
    - _2_ Plasma [HCO_3^-] is decreased.
    - _3_ CSF HCO_3^- diffuses into the blood.
    - _8_ pH is normalized.
    - _1_ Buffering of increased plasma [H^+] begins.
    - _4_ CSF pH decreases.
    - _7_ Plasma PCO_2 and [H_2CO_3] is decreased.
    - _6_ Ventilation increases.

21. The "standard bicarbonate" procedure is based on the assumption that:
    A. Abnormal PCO_2 does not affect plasma [HCO_3^-] in acid-base disturbances.
    B. [HCO_3^-] does not change with changes in the respiratory acid-base component.
    C. Abnormal [HCO_3^-] with a PCO_2 of 40 mm Hg indicates a metabolic acid-base disturbance.
    D. Intravascular and extravascular gas diffusion occurring in acid-base changes occurs in the laboratory.

22. A *positive* base excess value means that a blood sample was titrated in the laboratory:
    A. With base to normalize pH
    B. With acid to normalize pH
    C. By removing dissolved CO_2 to normalize pH
    D. By equilibrating blood PCO_2 with room air PCO_2

23. If [HCO_3^-] is constant, an increase in PCO_2 from 40 to 55 mm Hg decreases a normal pH (7.40) to:
    A. 6.95
    B. 7.355
    C. 7.31
    D. 6.5

II. Assessment and Treatment of Hypoxia

24. All of the following are signs of acute hypoxemia *except:*
    A. Tachycardia
    B. Mild hypertension
    C. Hypotension
    D. Hypoventilation

25. Hypoxic hypoxia is distinguished from all other types of hypoxia by the:
    A. Mean P_AO_2
    B. PaO_2
    C. CaO_2
    D. Way it responds to higher F_IO_2s

26. Anemic hypoxia differs from other hypoxias in that its primary defect is associated with:
    A. The relationship between P_AO_2 and PaO_2
    B. Oxygen carrying capacity
    C. Blood flow
    D. The diffusion pathway

27. *Primary* treatment for the cause of stagnant hypoxia is aimed at:
    A. Increasing functional hemoglobin levels
    B. Improving ventilation
    C. Restoring blood flow
    D. Increasing F_IO_2

28. *Acute* hypoxemia normally stimulates all of the following responses *except*:
    A. Increased cardiac output
    B. Improved tissue perfusion
    C. Increased erythrocyte production
    D. Increased minute ventilation

29. A standing, 70-year-old person normally has a PaO_2 ($\pm$ 12 mm Hg) of:
    A. 74 mm Hg
    B. 79 mm Hg
    C. 85 mm Hg
    D. 90 mm Hg

30. An individual's sea level PaO_2 = 95 mm Hg. At a barometric pressure of 720 mm Hg, the PaO_2 is:
    A. 100 mm Hg
    B. 94 mm Hg
    C. 90 mm Hg
    D. 85 mm Hg

31. A general "rule of thumb" is that at sea level, an additional 10% F_IO_2 will increase PaO_2 by approximately:
    A. 50 mm Hg
    B. 10 mm Hg
    C. 76 mm Hg
    D. 47 mm Hg

32. As the degree of shunt increases, the effectiveness of oxygen therapy (increases, decreases).

III. Treatment of Hypoxemia and Shunting

33. Risk for retinopathy of prematurity in the newborn is best determined by monitoring:
    A. PaO_2
    B. CaO_2
    C. F_IO_2
    D. SaO_2

34. Oxygen therapy is effective in treating all of the following *except:*
    A. $\dot{V}_A/\dot{Q}_C$ mismatch
    B. Absolute shunting
    C. Diffusion defects
    D. Hypoventilation

35. Which of the following is true of positive end-expiratory pressure (PEEP)?
    A. It increases intrapulmonary shunt.
    B. It increases lung compliance.
    C. It decreases FRC.
    D. It decreases transpulmonary pressure.

36. Disease states normally treated with continuous positive airway pressure (CPAP) and PEEP include all of the following *except:*
    A. Adult respiratory distress syndrome
    B. Alveolar instability secondary to surfactant abnormalities
    C. Extensive intrapulmonary shunting
    D. Lobar alveolar collapse

37. The permissive hypercapnia mechanical ventilation strategy includes:
    A. Pressure-controlled ventilation (maximum pressure is limited)
    B. Larger-than-normal tidal volumes
    C. Mechanical ventilation-induced alkalosis
    D. Variable breath-to-breath inspiratory alveolar pressures

38. Inverse ratio ventilation improves oxygenation because:
    A. Peak inspiratory pressure increases
    B. Mean alveolar pressure increases
    C. Expiratory time increases
    D. The inspiratory/expiratory ratio decreases

▶ Putting It All Together

1. A patient with chronic obstructive pulmonary disease has a pH of 7.37, a $PaCO_2$ of 55 mm Hg, and a $[HCO_3^-]$ of 31 mEq/L. Classify the acid-base condition.

2. Days later, the same patient develops a respiratory infection and presents with the following arterial blood gas analysis: pH = 7.43, PCO_2 = 48, and $[HCO_3^-]$ = 31 mEq/L. What is your interpretation?

3. In what way does hypoxemia cause respiratory alkalosis? What are the acid-base consequences of prolonged (i.e., several days) hypoxemia? What are the immediate acid-base consequences of correcting prolonged hypoxemia (will hyperventilation persist)?

4. A patient with fibrotic lung disease has poor alveolar-capillary membrane oxygen diffusion. The patient is chronically hypoxemic (PaO_2 = 57 mm Hg and SaO_2 = 88%) while breathing room air and has a hemoglobin concentration of 17 g/dl. Calculate the arterial oxygen content; state whether or not it is abnormal; and discuss the reason for the patient's arterial oxygen content.

5. Arterial blood gases for your patient are: PaO_2 = 57 mm Hg, $PaCO_2$ = 38 mm Hg, SaO_2 = 88%, $[HCO_3^-]$ = 24, pH = 7.4, and Hb = 12 g/dl. Cardiac output is 4.8 L/min. Calculate the oxygen delivery rate and oxygen extraction ratio (assuming normal resting oxygen consumption = 250 mL/min). What corrective action will yield the most immediate improvement in the patient's oxygen delivery?

6. Arterial blood gas samples are usually drawn during cardiopulmonary resuscitation (CPR) in hospital settings while the cardiac arrest victim is being aggressively hyperventilated with 100% oxygen and receiving chest compressions. These blood gas samples sometimes have pH levels < 7.2, PCO_2s < 30 mm Hg, $[HCO_3^-]$s < 12 mEq/L, and normal to high PO_2s. Identify the acid-base and oxygenation disturbances and why they occur under these conditions.

▷ Cases To Consider

1. A patient with chronic obstructive pulmonary disease with chronic hypercapnia is receiving mechanical ventilation for respiratory failure. Arterial blood gases examined immediately before intubation indicated the following: pH = 7.25, PaO_2 = 45 mm Hg, $PaCO_2$ = 80 mm Hg, and $[HCO_3^-]$ = 34 mEq/L. You obtain a second arterial blood gas 30 minutes after the start of mechanical ventilation. The new results are: pH = 7.35, PaO_2 = 80 mm Hg, $PaCO_2$ = 64 mm Hg, and $[HCO_3^-]$ = 34 mEq/L. Concerned that the current ventilator settings are inappropriate because of the high $PaCO_2$, the attending physician asks whether the patient's breathing frequency or tidal volume should be increased. What is your answer? What are the implications of increasing alveolar ventilation at this point?

2. An elderly asthmatic patient is brought to the clinic in acute respiratory distress. She has had the "flu" for 2 days and indicates that she has had diarrhea since her symptoms began. She is wheezing audibly, very short of breath, and speaks in broken sentences. She now states that she ran out of her bronchodilator medication 3 days ago. An arterial blood gas analysis performed while the patient is breathing room air reveals a PO_2 of 55 mm Hg, PCO_2 of 47 mm Hg, pH of 7.25, and $[HCO_3^-]$ of 20 mEq/L. A repeat blood gas after supplemental oxygen is given at 2 L/min by nasal cannula shows that PO_2 has improved to 90 mm Hg. Classify the patient's acid-base disturbance and its cause. Identify the ventilation/perfusion defect responsible for the low PO_2. What therapy(ies) will immediately address her acid-base and oxygenation problems? Why?

Section II
The Cardiovascular System

Chapter 14

Functional Anatomy of the Cardiovascular System

▷ Points to Remember

- Cardiovascular and pulmonary functions are inextricably linked and are vital to tissue oxygenation.
- The four chambers of the heart are the two collecting chambers (atria) and the two pumping chambers (ventricles).
- Back flow of blood into the atria from ventricles during systole is prevented by the tricuspid (right) and mitral (left) valves.
- Pulmonary and aortic valves prevent back flow of blood into the ventricles during diastole.
- The major heart sounds are produced by forceful closure of the heart's valves.
- Cardiac muscle perfusion occurs during ventricular diastole.
- Very high heart rates decrease diastolic time and ventricular filling time, reducing coronary vessel perfusion and ventricular stroke volume.
- The conducting fibers of the AV node normally slow cardiac impulse transmission, preventing high ventricular rates.
- Cardiac muscle oxygenation is blood flow dependent because of the high oxygen extraction ratio and a lack of collateral circulation.
- Cardiac muscle mass functions as a syncytium (single muscle fiber); stimulating one muscle fiber causes all muscle fibers to contract.
- Stretching the muscle fibers of the heart increases their force of contraction (Frank-Starling mechanism); thus the heart is able to adjust its stroke volume from minute-to-minute.
- In the arterial vascular system, distensible arteries and high resistance arterioles change intermittent left ventricular flow into continuous capillary flow.

- Capillary diameter is dependent on intravascular volume and pressure.
- Most of the total blood volume is in the venous system, which is a very distensible and low pressure system.
- Venovasoconstriction moves large volumes of venous blood into the arterial circulation during shock states.
- Arterial blood pressure is determined by stroke volume, vascular resistance, and blood volume.

▶ The Basics

I. The Heart

1. Beginning inside the heart and moving outward, number the following features of the heart in order.
   _____ Pericardial fluid
   _____ Parietal pericardium
   _____ Ventricle
   _____ Myocardium
   _____ Epicardium
   _____ Fibrous pericardium
   _____ Endocardium

2. The point of maximal impact (PMI) is palpable at the level of the:
   A. Second intercostal space at the midsternal line
   B. Second intercostal space at the midclavicular line
   C. Fifth intercostal space at the midclavicular line
   D. Fifth intercostal space at the midaxillary line

3. The right ventricle is positioned (anterior, posterior) to the left ventricle.

4. Number the following structures sequentially as they are encountered by the blood. Begin at the systemic venous side of the heart.
   _____ Left ventricle
   _____ Right ventricle
   _____ Left atrium
   _____ Right atrium
   _____ Pulmonic valve
   _____ Tricuspid valve
   _____ Aortic valve
   _____ Bicuspid valve
   _____ Vena cavae
   _____ Pulmonary artery
   _____ Aorta
   _____ Lungs

5. All of the following are true of the left ventricle *except:*
   A. It has a spherical cross-section.
   B. It wraps around the right ventricle.
   C. It pumps against higher resistance than the right ventricle.
   D. It has a greater muscle mass than the right ventricle.

6. Match the description on the right with the appropriate term on the left.
   _____ Trabeculae carneae
   _____ Chordae tendineae
   _____ Myocardium
   _____ Foramen ovale
   _____ Papillary muscles
   _____ Fibrous annuli
   _____ Pericardial fluid
   _____ Visceral pericardium

   A. Epicardium
   B. Forms the bulk of the heart wall
   C. Muscle bundles on ventricular inner surface
   D. Allows frictionless cardiac movement
   E. Cone-shaped pillars
   F. Tethers that prevent atrioventricular valvular regurgitation
   G. Small depression in the interatrial septum
   H. Connected-ring framework to which muscle and valves are attached

7. Coronary arteries receive blood directly from the:
   A. Left ventricle
   B. Aorta
   C. Pulmonary trunk
   D. Left atrium

8. Myocardial perfusion occurs during ventricular (diastole, systole).

9. Deoxygenated blood that causes a normal right-to-left anatomic shunt flows into the left atrium through the:
   A. Thebesian veins
   B. Coronary sinus
   C. Pulmonary veins
   D. Coronary arteries

10. Myocardial ischemia is the direct result of:
    A. Myocardial tissue death
    B. Angina pectoris
    C. Coronary artery occlusion
    D. Coronary artery vasodilation

11. The myocardial oxygen extraction rate at rest is approximately:
    A. 25%
    B. 30%
    C. 65%
    D. 70%

12. Label the features of the cardiac conduction system on the illustration below: left ventricle, Purkinje fibers, left atrium, apex, interventricular septum, left and right bundle branches, atrioventricular node, sinoatrial node, and atrioventricular bundle.

A. _____

B. _____

C. _____

D. _____

E. _____

F. _____

G. _____

H. _____

I. _____

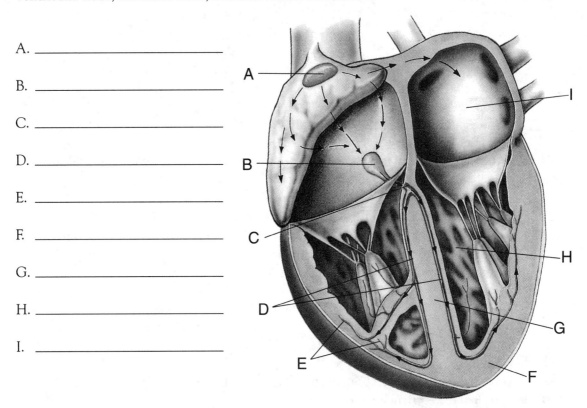

(Art from Seeley RR, Stephens TD, Tate P: *Anatomy and physiology*, ed 3, New York 1995, McGraw-Hill.)

13. Electrical impulses that stimulate ventricular contraction are initiated by the:
    A. SA node
    B. AV bundle
    C. Purkinje fibers
    D. Intranodal pathway

14. The electrical connection between atrial and ventricular muscle is the:
    A. AV bundle
    B. Intranodal pathway
    C. Purkinje fibers
    D. AV node

15. Before transmitting to the ventricles, electrical impulses are slowed by the:
    A. AV bundle
    B. AV node
    C. SA node
    D. Purkinje fibers

16. All of the following are true of parasympathetic fibers *except*:
    A. Their stimulation slows heart rate.
    B. Their stimulation decreases myocardial force of contraction.
    C. They are mainly beta-1 type fibers.
    D. They are mainly distributed to atrial muscle and nodes.

17. Match the appropriate description on the right with each property of cardiac muscle on the left.
    _____ Muscle fiber   A. Basic contractile unit
    _____ Sarcolemma   B. Thin myofilaments
    _____ T-tubule   C. Thick myofilaments
    _____ Sarcoplasmic reticulum D. Muscle cell
    _____ Myofibril   E. Protein disk-like structure
    _____ Myosin   F. Interconnected network of canals
    _____ Actin parallel to T-tubules G. Formed by numerous sarcomeres
    _____ Sarcomere   H. Formed by sarcolemma dipping into muscle fiber
    _____ Z-line joined end-to-end I. Muscle cell membrane

18. Number the following steps as they occur in excitation and contraction of muscle fibers.
    _____ Acetylcholine stimulates the sarcolemma.
    _____ Tropomyosin strands slide into actin grooves.
    _____ Myosin cross-bridges pull the actin filament toward the sarcomere's center.
    _____ ATP molecules bind with the myosin cross-bridge and pull it to its resting position.
    _____ Sarcoplasmic reticulum releases Ca^{++} ions.
    _____ Energized myosin cross-bridges bind with actin sites.

19. The Frank-Starling law of the heart asserts that the force of cardiac contraction is:
    A. Indirectly proportional to the number of cross bridges formed between actin and myosin filaments
    B. Proportional to end-systolic pressure
    C. Proportional to post-contraction length of cardiac muscle fiber
    D. Proportional to ventricular preload

20. The average time measured from the beginning of systole to the end of diastole is approximately:
    A. 0.4 seconds
    B. 0.5 seconds
    C. 0.8 seconds
    D. 1.2 seconds

21. Normally, resting ventricular contraction ejects blood volume equal to:
    A. 70 ml
    B. 80 ml
    C. 90 ml
    D. 100 ml

22. The normal resting ventricular ejection fraction is approximately:
    A. 50%
    B. 60%
    C. 75%
    D. 80%

II. The Vascular System

23. Match the term on the left with the correct description on the right.
    _____ Left ventricle
    _____ Conducting arteries
    _____ Arterioles
    _____ Microcirculation
    _____ Anastomosis
    _____ Veins
    _____ Pulse pressure

    A. Resistance vessels with major influence on blood pressure and flow
    B. Contain approximately 64% of total blood volume
    C. Capillary beds
    D. Systemic pump
    E. Difference between systolic and diastolic values
    F. Direct arteriovenous connection
    G. Largest, high-pressure systemic vessels

24. Precapillary sphincters normally decrease blood flow in response to:
    A. Tissue hypoxia
    B. Low metabolic activity
    C. Strenuous exercise
    D. Low tissue blood flow needs

25. Venous return to the heart occurs through all the following mechanisms *except*:
    A. Sympathetic venous vasodilation
    B. "Cardiac suction" during cardiac pumping action
    C. Muscular "milking" of leg veins
    D. Subatmospheric thoracic pressures during breathing

26. Estimated mean arterial pressure (MAP) is calculated as:
    A. (Systolic pressure + Diastolic pressure) / 2
    B. [2 x (Systolic pressure + Diastolic pressure)] / 3
    C. (Systolic pressure + 2 x Diastolic pressure) / 3
    D. (Systolic pressure + Diastolic pressure) / 3

27. If the MAP is 110 mm Hg, right atrial pressure is 6 mm Hg, and cardiac output is 4 L/min, systemic vascular resistance (SVR) is:
    A. 29 mm Hg/L/min
    B. 73 mm Hg/L/min
    C. 26 mm Hg/L/min
    D. 31 mm Hg/L/min

28. If SVR increases, left ventricular afterload (increases, decreases).

29. If the MAP and right atrial pressure (RAP) remain constant while SVR decreases, cardiac output will (increase, decrease).

30. Normal RAP is approximately:
    A. 0 mm Hg
    B. 10 mm Hg
    C. 12 mm Hg
    D. 25 mm Hg

31. Venous blood flow increases in the presence of:
    A. Arterial vasodilation
    B. Decreased blood volume
    C. Increased RAP
    D. Decreased venous tone

32. Mechanisms for local control of blood flow includes all of the following *except*:
    A. Increased metabolic rate
    B. Hypoxemia
    C. Increased nitric oxide release
    D. Sympathetic release of norepinephrine

33. Minute-to-minute blood pressure is regulated by the:
    A. Renin-angiotensin-aldosterone mechanism
    B. Carotid and aortic baroreceptors
    C. Release of antidiuretic hormone
    D. Release of atrial natriuretic hormone

▶ Putting It All Together

1. Left ventricular afterload is normally decreased by:
   A. Increased blood viscosity
   B. Decreased arteriole sphincter tone
   C. Atherosclerosis
   D. Increased blood volume

2. Number the following events of the cardiac cycle. Assume that the cycle begins with ventricular contraction.
   _____ Ventricular pressures rise enough to open semilunar valves.
   _____ The ventricles contract against closed semilunar valves.
   _____ Ventricular pressures build, forcefully closing the atrioventricular valves.
   _____ Atrial pressures fall as blood drains into the ventricles.
   _____ Back flow of blood into ventricles is stopped abruptly, causing dilation and recoil of the aorta and pulmonary artery.
   _____ The ventricles relax; their pressures fall; and semilunar valves snap shut.
   _____ Ventricular contraction closes the atrioventricular valves.
   _____ The ejection period occurs.
   _____ The atria contract, slightly distending ventricular walls.
   _____ Ventricular pressures fall and atrioventricular valves open.

3. Using your answers from the previous question, indicate during which events the following are present.
   _____ A. Dicrotic notch (in aortic and pulmonary artery waveforms)
   _____ B. First heart sound
   _____ C. Second heart sound
   _____ D. Isovolumetric contraction
   _____ E. Isovolumetric relaxation
   _____ F. Atrial kick

4. Why is sympathetic peripheral vasoconstriction beneficial to central organs in hypovolemic shock?

5. Discuss why peripheral edema occurs in right ventricular failure.

6. Bradycardia is most likely to occur during which of the following:
   A. Exercise
   B. Administration of catecholamine drugs
   C. Tracheal suctioning
   D. Anxiety

7. Identify the mechanism responsible for causing bradycardia in your selection for Question 6.

8. Jugular venous distension, pedal edema, and abdominal ascites are relieved in patients receiving diuretic medication. Why are these abnormalities present? Why does a diuretic drug relieve them?

9. Normal urine production rate depends, in part, on adequate perfusion. What is the impact of left ventricular failure on urine output? Why?

▶ Cases to Consider

1. You are called to assess a patient brought to the emergency room in obvious respiratory distress. While exercising, the patient experienced sudden pain in the right upper chest. Since then, the patient has been very short of breath, hypoxemic, and tachycardic. The patient's medical history includes bullous emphysema (emphysema with abnormally large, thin-walled spaces in the lung parenchyma). As you auscultate the patient's chest, you hear no breath sounds over the right upper chest and notice that the patient's point of maximal impact (PMI) is shifted laterally to the patient's left. Current blood pressure readings are reduced from the patient's baseline values. An electrocardiogram (ECG) indicates only right ventricular hypertrophy, which is consistent with previous ECGs for this patient. Realizing the gravity of the situation, you immediately insert a large bore needle into an intercostal space on the patient's right chest wall. You state to the caregivers that this measure will relieve the patient's respiratory distress, hypoxemia, tachycardia, and poor blood pressure. Justify your action by stating why it will improve each of the patient's abnormal signs. Why is the subsequent placement of a chest tube attached to a vacuum necessary?

2. You are caring for a chronic obstructive pulmonary disease patient in the intensive care unit. A Swan-Ganz catheter has been placed in the patient's pulmonary artery to monitor hemodynamic status. The patient currently exhibits pedal edema and jugular venous distension (JVD). Central venous pressure (CVP) is 16 mm Hg. Reviewing the patient's chart, you notice that the patient's home medications include a maintenance dose of furosemide, a diuretic. The patient's current hospital medication list does not include any drugs with diuretic effects. You also note a weight gain of 4 pounds since admission yesterday. You contact the critical care physician to get this patient started on a diuretic medication. Other than the fact that this medication was used at home, what reasons will you give for adding it at this time?

Chapter 15
Cardiac Electrophysiology

▷ Points To Remember

- Membrane potential is the difference in the electrical charge between ion concentrations immediately inside and outside the cardiac cell membrane.
- Outward diffusion of intracellular potassium (K^+) along its concentration gradient creates a negative resting membrane potential (RMP).
- Depolarizing stimuli cause the RMP to become less negative until threshold potential (TP) is reached.
- At TP, sodium (Na^+) rushes into the cell and depolarizes the cell membrane.
- The action potential is a recording of transmembrane voltage over time during depolarization and repolarization.
- The action potential plateau phase occurs when calcium (Ca^{++}) flows into the cell, prolonging depolarization and facilitating muscle contraction.
- Propagation of the action potential throughout the entire heart occurs through highly permeable cardiac cell membranes called intercalated disks.
- Extracellular K^+ and Ca^{++} concentrations affect depolarization characteristics of the cardiac fiber.
- Entry of Ca^{++} into the cardiac cell can be either enhanced or blocked by cardiac drugs, affecting depolarization and muscle contraction characteristics.
- The heart's spontaneous pacemaker, the sino-atrial (SA) node, depolarizes cyclicly at a rate higher than that of any other cardiac fiber.
- Ectopic pacemakers (pacemakers other than the SA node) cause premature beats if the SA node is suppressed or if other foci (focal points) become more excitable.
- The cardiac conduction system rapidly transmits the SA node impulse throughout the atria and ventricles.
- The SA node impulse is delayed slightly by the atrioventricular (AV) node, allowing adequate ventricular filling time.
- Sympathetic stimulation increases the heart rate and force of contraction; parasympathetic stimulation does the opposite.

▷ The Basics

I. Membrane Potentials

1. Cardiac muscle cells maintain high concentrations of (positive, negative) ions outside and (positive, negative) ions inside their cell membranes.

2. The resting membrane potential (RMP) is the difference in the electrical charge between:
   A. Ions outside the cell membrane
   B. Both sides of the cell membrane
   C. Ions inside the cell membrane
   D. Opposing ends of the cardiac muscle fiber

3. Normal RMP of cardiac fibers is approximately:
   A. -25 to -35 mV
   B. -40 to -60 mV
   C. -70 to -75 mV
   D. -85 to -90 mV

4. The main ions involved in generating the RMP include all of the following *except*:
   A. Ca^{++}
   B. H^+
   C. K^+
   D. Na^+

5. A resting cardiac cell membrane is highly permeable to _____ ions but only slightly permeable to _____ and _____ ions.

6. Diffusion forces cause K^+ movement (into, out of) the cell; electrostatic attraction causes it to move (into, out of) the cell.

7. Extracellular K^+ ion concentration is approximately:
   A. 4 mEq/L
   B. 144 mEq/L
   C. 1 mEq/L
   D. 141 mEq/L

II. Ion Channels and Gates

8. Permeability of the myocardial cell membrane to Na^+ and K^+ is mainly controlled by:
   A. Voltage-sensitive gating proteins
   B. Leak channels
   C. Slow channels
   D. The Na^+ - K^+ pump

9. The electrical event in the myocardial cell that leads to muscle fiber contraction is called:
   A. The resting membrane potential
   B. Voltage gating
   C. Ion pumping
   D. The action potential

III. The Action Potential

10. On the following illustration, number the phases (0 through 4) of Na^+, K^+, and Ca^{++} movement as they occur during generation of the action potential. Then place the phase numbers in the appropriate positions on the action potential waveform.

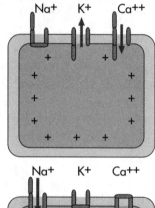
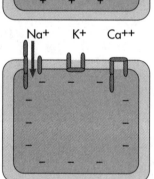
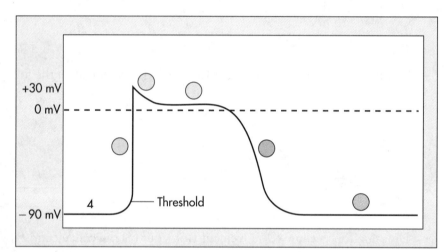
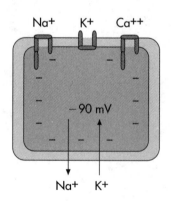
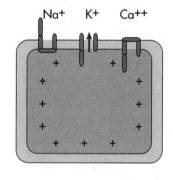
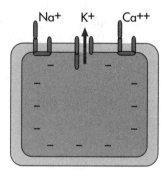

108   The Cardiovascular System

11. Match the letter of the statement on the right with the correct term on the left.
    _____ Depolarization
    _____ Repolarization
    _____ Action potential
    _____ Threshold potential
    _____ Refractory
    _____ Excitability
    _____ Hyperpolarized

    A. Muscle fiber characteristic during action potential phases 0 through 3
    B. Resting membrane potential changes to 0 mV
    C. All activation gates open, allowing rapid influx of Na^+
    D. Cardiac cell membrane less susceptible to depolarization
    E. Resting membrane potential changes to -90 mV
    F. Voltage plotted against time, depicting changes in membrane potential
    G. Difference between resting membrane and threshold potentials

12. *During* phase 0 of the action potential:
    A. The muscle fiber accepts a polarizing stimulus
    B. Cell membrane permeability to Na^+ increases up to 1,000 times
    C. K^+ flows out of the cell
    D. Na^+ is pumped out of the cell

13. Ca^{++} flows into the myocardial cell during phase:
    A. 0
    B. 1
    C. 2
    D. 3

14. The action potential phase that lasts the longest is the:
    A. Plateau phase
    B. Depolarization phase
    C. Repolarization phase
    D. Resting membrane phase

IV. Drugs, Extracellular Ion Concentration, and the Action Potential

15. On the voltage-time graph below, draw the relative positions of three action potentials as they appear in normal, hypokalemic, and hyperkalemic conditions.

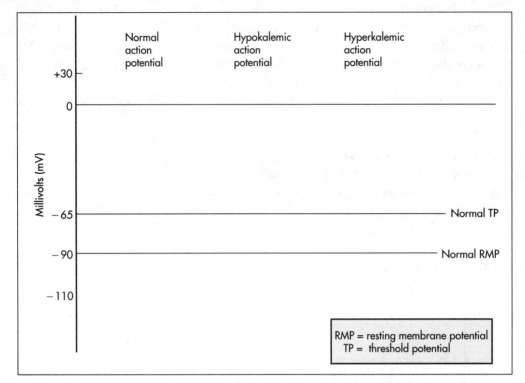

16. Match the statements on the left with those on the right. (Note: Letters may be used once, twice, or not at all.)

    _____ Cardiac cell membrane is more excitable
    _____ Cardiac cell membrane is less excitable
    _____ Amplitude of action potential is increased
    _____ Amplitude of action potential is reduced
    _____ Heart rate is increased
    _____ Heart rate is decreased
    _____ Stroke volume is increased
    _____ Stroke volume is decreased

    A. True of hyperkalemia
    B. True of hypokalemia
    C. Not true of hyperkalemia or hypokalemia

17. Hypocalcemia results in all of the following abnormalities *except*:
    A. Increased heart muscle excitability
    B. Higher resting membrane potential
    C. Lower threshold potential
    D. Na^+ channels open sooner during depolarization

18. Catecholamine drug action tends to:
    A. Reduce intracellular levels of AMP
    B. Enhance activation of Ca^{++} channels
    C. Decrease cardiac contractility
    D. Enhance parasympathetic stimulation

19. Calcium channel blockers result in all of the following *except:*
    A. Increased stroke volume
    B. Decreased oxygen consumption
    C. Coronary vasodilation
    D. Decreased muscle contractility

V. Rhythmic Excitation of the Heart

20. The ability of cardiac tissue to spontaneously depolarize is called _____. _____ describes the ability of cardiac tissue to spontaneously depolarize in a repetitive manner. The inclination to spontaneously depolarize is called _____. _____ is the ability cardiac muscle fibers have to shorten in length.

21. Cardiac tissue that generates the greatest frequency of impulses is called the:
    A. Bundle of His
    B. AV node
    C. SA node
    D. A-V bundle

22. The impulse for an ectopic beat must:
    A. Originate in the sinus node
    B. Depolarize fibers more slowly than impulses from the sinus node
    C. Originate from a pacemaker more excitable than SA fibers
    D. Conduct through the SA node

23. AV fibers have a spontaneous depolarization rate of:
    A. 15 to 40 beats/min
    B. 30 to 40 beats/min
    C. 40 to 60 beats/min
    D. 70 to 80 beats/min

VI. Transmission of Impulses Through the Heart

24. The impulse from the SA node reaches the left atrium through the:
    A. Bachmann's bundle
    B. Bundle of His
    C. Purkinje fibers
    D. A-V bundle

25. The AV nodal system consists of all of the following *except* the:
    A. Internodal pathways
    B. Junctional fibers
    C. AV node
    D. Bundle of His

26. Normal travel time for a depolarizing impulse is shortest:
    A. From the SA node to the last ventricular fiber
    B. From the SA node to the AV node
    C. Through the AV node
    D. Through bundle branches and Purkinje fibers

27. Parasympathetic-stimulated release of acetylcholine causes all of the following *except*:
    A. Decreased SA node firing rate
    B. Increased atrioventricular conduction rate
    C. Decreased AV node excitability
    D. AV heart block

28. Sympathetic stimulation has all of the following effects on cardiac function *except*:
    A. Increased cardiac fiber excitability
    B. Release of norepinephrine
    C. Increased fiber permeability to Na^+ and Ca^{++}
    D. Decreased SA node firing rate

▷ Putting It All Together

1. Describe the impact of an abnormally high AV conduction rate on cardiac output.

2. Some drugs used to treat pulmonary diseases are beta-agonists, that is, they stimulate beta receptor sites. What change in cardiac vital signs should be anticipated for a patient taking a drug that stimulates cardiac beta receptor sites?

3. In what way will the heart rate change in the presence of conduction abnormalities that prevent transmission of SA node impulses to the ventricles?

4. The rate of conduction over the Bachmann's bundle internodal pathway is higher than the conduction rate of most other atrial muscle fibers. What would occur if this conduction rate was equal to other atrial fibers?

5. Why should a calcium channel blocker not be given to a patient with low blood pressure?

6. What deleterious cardiac side effects are possible when using potassium-depleting diuretic drugs on patients?

▶ A Case to Consider

1. You are the respiratory care practitioner caring for a patient with chronic lung disease. When reviewing the patient's chart, you notice that, in addition to hyperinflation on the current chest x-ray, cardiomegaly (an enlarged heart) is also present. Visual inspection of the patient reveals edema over the abdomen and extremities. During your discussion with the patient's physician, the physician comments that she believes the patient has progressed to chronic congestive heart failure. She intends to begin diuretic therapy to relieve acute systemic venous congestion, but is concerned about the potassium-depleting effects of many diuretic drugs. You state that an inotropic drug, such as digitalis, may be helpful for her patient. Why is a drug such as digitalis beneficial in this situation? What is the primary mechanism of its inotropic action?

Chapter 16

The Electrocardiogram and Cardiac Arrhythmias

▷ Points To Remember

- Voltage changes during depolarization and repolarization of the heart generate waves and complexes of the electrocardiogram (ECG).
- Twelve different leads (electrode systems) provide twelve different perspectives on cardiac electrical activity.
- The ECG's polarity is determined by current flow direction relative to lead placement.
- Mean cardiac vector (mean direction of cardiac current flow) is determined by analyzing the ECG of different leads.
- Heart rate, conduction time, and abnormal arrhythmias are monitored by the ECG recording.
- Cardiac arrhythmias are caused by a number of factors: dilated, stretched muscle, electrolyte imbalances, pH changes, ischemia (tissue hypoxia), infarction (tissue death), abnormal sympathetic or parasympathetic tone, ingested stimulants (such as caffeine, tobacco, alcohol) and drugs.
- Treatment of arrhythmias must address underlying causes and concurrent symptoms.
- Ventricular fibrillation is the most life-threatening arrhythmia and must be treated with countershock (defibrillation).

▷ The Basics

I. The Normal Electrocardiogram

1. The ECG directly measures all of the following *except*:
   A. Depolarization time
   B. Voltage changes
   C. Force of contraction
   D. Repolarization time

2. On the following ECG tracing, label the P, Q, R, S, and T waves; the P-R and Q-T intervals; and the ST segment.

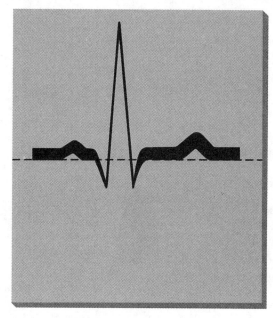

(Art from Thibodeau GA, Patton KT: *Anatomy and physiology,* ed 3, St Louis, 1996, Mosby.)

3. Match the components of the ECG on the left with the correct statements on the right. (Note: Each ECG component may have more than one correct statement, and some statements may not be needed.)

_____ P wave
_____ QRS complex
_____ T wave
_____ P-R interval
_____ ST segment
_____ Q-T interval

A. Produced by ventricular repolarization
B. Produced by atrial depolarization
C. Represents ventricular refractory period
D. Represents time required for SA node impulse to travel to ventricles
E. Represents ventricular conduction time
F. Represents early phase of ventricular repolarization
G. Associated with ventricular contraction
H. Produced by atrial repolarization
I. Associated with ventricular relaxation
J. Associated with atrial contraction

4. The normal P-R interval time is between:
   A. 0.12 and 0.20 sec
   B. 0.02 and 0.12 sec
   C. 0.20 and 0.24 sec
   D. 0.10 and 0.20 sec

5. Electrical current generated by depolarization in the heart flows from:
   A. Right to left
   B. Left to right
   C. Base to apex
   D. Apex to base

6. For the illustration below, draw ECGs for the bipolar and unipolar leads as indicated by the "+" signs, "−" signs, and dashed lines.

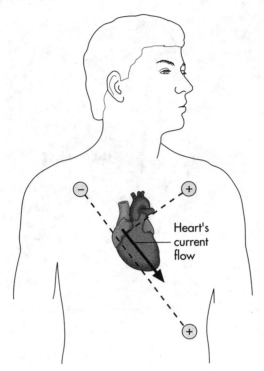

7. At standard recording speed, the small, 1 mm squares represent:
   A. 0.02 sec
   B. 0.04 sec
   C. 0.10 sec
   D. 0.20 sec

8. Within each large square on an ECG grid there are:
   A. 3 small squares
   B. 4 small squares
   C. 5 small squares
   D. 6 small squares

9. The upper edge of ECG paper has evenly spaced vertical lines representing time intervals of:
   A. 3 seconds
   B. 4 seconds
   C. 5 seconds
   D. 6 seconds

10. Einthoven's triangle is formed by three standard limb leads. In lead I, the negative electrode is placed on the _____ and the positive on the _____. Lead II electrodes are placed with the negative electrode on the _____ and the positive on the _____. In lead III, the negative electrode is placed on the _____ and the positive on the _____.

11. Einthoven discovered that the amplitude of the QRS complex recorded in lead _____ is always equal to the sum of the voltages in leads _____ and _____.

116 The Cardiovascular System

12. Frontal plane leads include all of the following *except*:
    A. Unipolar limb leads
    B. Augmented limb leads
    C. Bipolar leads
    D. Precordial leads

13. On the illustration below, label the following: 0°, -90°, +90°, aV_R, aV_F, aV_L, lead I, lead II, lead III, and the normal cardiac vector.

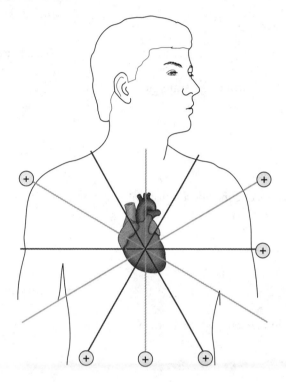

14. All of the following are factors that cause electrical axis deviations *except*:
    A. Bundle branch conduction block
    B. Myocardial infarction
    C. Change in heart position
    D. Uniform hypertrophy of both ventricles

15. List the four steps to systematic ECG analysis.

16. Regularity of ventricular rhythm is determined from a beat-to-beat comparison of:
    A. P-R intervals
    B. R-R intervals
    C. Q-T intervals
    D. R-S intervals

17. Ventricular rhythm is irregular if the time interval between beats varies by more than:
    A. 0.02 sec
    B. 0.04 sec
    C. 0.16 sec
    D. 0.20 sec

18. Match each ECG abnormality on the left with the appropriate cardiac activity on the right.
    _____ More P waves than QRS complexes
    _____ P wave polarity opposite of expected
    _____ Wide QRS complex
    _____ P wave follows QRS complex
    _____ PR interval greater than 0.2 sec
    _____ Two QRS complexes of different polarity

    A. Slowed SA node-ventricular impulse conduction
    B. Not all atrial impulses are conducted to ventricles
    C. Slowed ventricular conduction velocity
    D. Presence of ectopic focus
    E. Impulse may originate in the AV node
    F. Atrial pacemaker site has changed

19. Normal sinus rhythm occurs when the sinus node initiates depolarizing impulses at a rate of:
    A. 80 to 100/min
    B. 80 to 120/min
    C. 60 to 100/min
    D. 60 to 80/min

20. Sinus tachycardia in adults occurs when a normally initiated and conducted heart rate is greater than:
    A. 90 beats/min
    B. 100 beats/min
    C. 110 beats/min
    D. 120 beats/min

21. Sinus bradycardia in adults occurs when a normally initiated and conducted heart rate is less than:
    A. 40 beats/min
    B. 50 beats/min
    C. 60 beats/min
    D. 70 beats/min

22. Premature atrial contractions may alter a normal ECG in all of the following ways *except*:
    A. Widened QRS complexes
    B. Irregularly spaced QRS complexes
    C. Abnormally shaped P waves
    D. P waves superimposed on T waves

23. Match the statement on the right with the term it describes on the left.
    _____ Atrial flutter
    _____ Atrial fibrillation
    _____ Junctional escape rhythm
    _____ Premature junctional contraction
    _____ Junctional tachycardia
    _____ Paroxysmal supraventricular tachycardia

    A. Caused by an irritable ectopic focus in junctional fibers
    B. In the absence of SA node impulses, firing rate is 40 to 60/min
    C. Caused by supraventricular pacemaker firing at 240 to 360 beats/min
    D. Junctional fibers generate a heart rate greater than 60 beats/min
    E. Junctional fibers generate bursts of heart rates up to 240 beats/min
    F. Uncoordinated discharge from ectopic atrial foci at a rate of 300 to 600/min

24. One characteristic of a junctional rhythm is:
    A. A firing rate higher than in normal sinus rhythm
    B. Abnormal QRS complexes
    C. A P-R interval longer than 12 seconds
    D. Abnormal P waves

25. A premature ventricular contraction (PVC) is initiated by an ectopic focus originating below the level of the:
    A. Sinoatrial node
    B. Atrial tissue
    C. Atrioventricular junctional fibers
    D. Branching point of the bundle of His

26. Characteristics of PVCs include all of the following *except*:
    A. PVCs occur prematurely.
    B. Normal heart rhythm is maintained.
    C. T waves of abnormal polarity are generated.
    D. The QRS complex is wide.

27. Match the terms on the left with the statements on the right.
    _____ Torsades de pointes
    _____ Ventricular fibrillation
    _____ Bigeminy
    _____ Ventricular tachycardia
    _____ Multifocal PVCs
    _____ Circus re-entry

    A. QRSs rhythmically change between positive and negative polarity
    B. Three or more PVCs in a row
    C. Fibrillatory pattern in which part of the heart muscle repolarizes before the rest finishes depolarizing
    D. Ventricles are a quivering, nonfunctional muscle mass
    E. Ectopic foci exist in different areas of the ventricles
    F. A PVC alternates every other beat with normal QRS

28. Type II second-degree AV heart block is characterized by:
    A. Constant P-R intervals and variable conduction ratios
    B. Complete blockage of SA node impulses to the ventricles
    C. Gradual lengthening of P-R intervals until a QRS fails to appear after a P wave
    D. Ventricular conduction of all SA node impulses; P-R intervals are greater than 0.2 seconds

29. In third degree AV heart block:
    A. Atrioventricular conduction rates are variable
    B. Sinus node impulses do not reach the ventricles
    C. The conduction ratio is 1:1, but conduction time is slowed
    D. The conduction ratio is variable, but conduction time is constant

30. A ventricular escape rhythm may exhibit all of the following *except*:
    A. Wider-than-normal QRS complexes
    B. Normal polarity QRS complexes
    C. A constant P wave-to-QRS conduction ratio
    D. Decreased cardiac output and blood pressure

▶ Putting It All Together

1. A patient's ECG records a negative QRS deflection in lead I and in lead aV_F. Assuming correct lead placement on this patient, comment on the heart's electrical axis.

2. If the heart rhythm is regular and the interval between two QRS complexes is three large ECG squares, what is the heart rate?
    A. 300 beats/min
    B. 150 beats/min
    C. 100 beats/min
    D. 75 beats/min

3. If the heart rhythm is irregular and the number of QRS complexes during two intervals marked by the vertical lines at the top of the ECG grid is 9, what is the heart rate?
    A. 45 beats/min
    B. 68 beats/min
    C. 90 beats/min
    D. 135 beats/min

4. In what way is cardiac output affected by the heart's mechanical activity when retrograde P waves are present on an ECG?

5. An ECG shows fine fibrillatory waves ("f" waves), no P waves, and a heart rate of 50 beats/min. All QRS complexes are widened and are of similar shape. Two types of arrhythmias are present. What are they? How many pacemakers are producing the QRS complexes, and what is the location of the pacemaker(s)?

6. In a condition called situs inversus, organs of the abdomen and thorax are reversed laterally. If the heart is transpositioned, but otherwise normal, in what way is the cardiac axis affected?

7. Even though both are very serious ventricular arrhythmias, why does ventricular fibrillation immediately have greater deleterious consequences than ventricular tachycardia?

8. A ventricular pacemaker located close to the bifurcation of the bundle of His produces a QRS complex similar to a normal complex. An impulse originating lower in the ventricles produces a wide, unusually shaped QRS. Why is this so?

9. What do conduction voltage and conduction time measurements on an ECG have in common and in what way do they differ?

▷ Cases to Consider

1. You are caring for a patient just admitted to your medical center's intensive care unit. This elderly man is being observed for unexplained syncope and hypotension. During your chart review, you note that the patient's normal weight is 80 kilograms, his heart rate is usually 90 to 110 beats/min, and he has been previously diagnosed with "mild" congestive heart failure. Assessing the patient, you find that his blood pressure remains low and his weight is 81 kilograms. An ECG monitor in the patient's room reveals normal QRS complexes with a very irregular rhythm. No P waves are present on the ECG, but QRS complexes are connected by a fine, irregular, "wavy" baseline. Between eight and nine QRS complexes are present in each 3-second interval on a printout of the ECG. The intensivist on duty asks for your conclusions on how this patient's condition evolved and any therapy you believe is indicated. How do you respond?

2. A patient being treated in the emergency department is being monitored by continuous ECG. A practitioner summons you to the bedside to observe the rhythm displayed on the ECG monitor. The practitioner believes that the patient should be given intravenous lidocaine to treat the rhythm. The monitor reveals only wide QRS complexes and P waves that do not associate with the QRS complexes. The heart rate is 45 to 50 beats/min. What arrhythmia is present? Do you concur with the suggested treatment?

Chapter 17

Control of Cardiac Output and Hemodynamics

▷ Points To Remember

- Cardiac output and venous return are interdependent; factors affecting one are important to the other.
- Stroke volume is determined by preload, afterload, and contractility.
- Preload is the load or stretch placed on myocardial fibers just before contraction.
- Afterload is the force opposing ejection of ventricular stroke volume.
- Contractility is the force of myocardial muscle fiber contraction at a given preload and afterload.
- Right atrial pressure (RAP) and pulmonary capillary wedge pressure (PCWP) are clinical indicators of right and left ventricular preload, respectively.
- Pulmonary vascular resistance (PVR) and systemic vascular resistance (SVR) are clinical indicators of right and left ventricular afterload, respectively.
- Right ventricular stroke work index (RVSWI) and left ventricular stroke work index (LVSWI) are indicators of right and left ventricular contractility, respectively.
- The cardiac and vascular function curves illustrate the interdependence of cardiac output and preload.
- The cardiac function curve is affected by preload, afterload, and contractility.
- The vascular function curve is affected by blood volume, vessel diameter, and vessel compliance.
- Regulatory factors in venous return and cardiac output are simultaneously resolved at a RAP of approximately 2 mm Hg and a cardiac output of 5 L/min.
- Hemodynamic measurements from a pulmonary artery catheter help quantify and monitor factors that affect cardiac and vascular performance.
- A ventricular function curve assists in classifying hemodynamic status into four distinct diagnostic subsets.

▶ The Basics

I. Factors Controlling Cardiac Output

1. Cardiac factors affecting cardiac output include all of the following *except*:
   A. Stretch of myocardial fibers just before contraction
   B. Arteriolar resistance
   C. Ventricular outflow resistance
   D. The force of myocardial fiber contraction

2. Ventricular preload is equal to:
   A. Ventricular end-systolic pressure
   B. Mean aortic pressure
   C. Ventricular end-diastolic pressure
   D. Mean systemic pressure

3. Of the following, the normal heart's pumping effectiveness is affected most by mean:
   A. Atrial pressure
   B. Pulmonary artery pressure
   C. Aortic pressure
   D. Systemic pressure

4. All of the following are clinical indicators of ventricular afterload *except*:
   A. Mean aortic pressure
   B. Mean pulmonary artery pressure
   C. End-diastolic pressure
   D. Vascular resistance

5. A clinical indicator of contractility is:
   A. Systemic vascular resistance
   B. Atrial pressure
   C. Mean pulmonary artery pressure
   D. Ventricular stroke work index

6. Decreased contractility is normally associated with:
   A. Above normal stroke volumes in the physiologic range
   B. Increased ejection fraction
   C. Increased ventricular preload
   D. Negative inotropic factors

7. On the vascular function graphs below, draw vascular function curves representing changes in venous return (and cardiac output) in the presence of hypervolemia and hypovolemia (graph "A") and increased and decreased vascular resistance (graph "B"). On graph "C," draw in the changes in the position of the cardiac function curve under conditions of increased and decreased cardiac contractility.

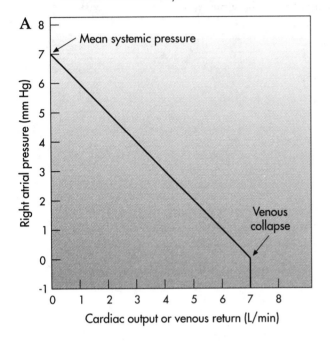
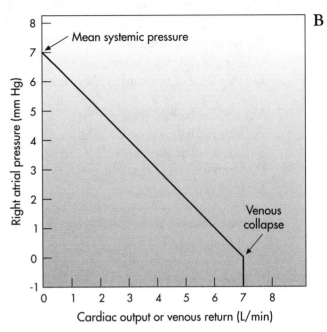
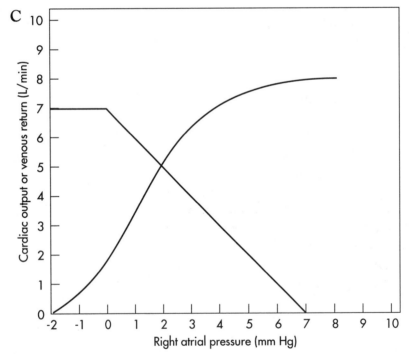

8. An acute decrease in myocardial contractility will cause venous return to:
   A. Decrease, then return to normal
   B. Decrease
   C. Increase, then return to normal
   D. Increase

9. An acute change in blood volume does not cause a change in:
   A. Cardiac output
   B. Venous return
   C. Contractility
   D. Right atrial pressure

10. Normally, increased arteriolar resistance results in:
    A. Decreased afterload
    B. Decreased preload
    C. Increased arterial pressure
    D. Increased cardiac output

11. Compensatory mechanisms for acute heart pumping failure include all of the following *except*:
    A. Improved contractility
    B. Vasodilation
    C. Sympathetic stimulation
    D. Renal fluid retention

II. Hemodynamic Measurements

12. Indicate the normal ranges for the following hemodynamic measurements.
Central venous pressure: _____
Pulmonary artery pressure (systolic/diastolic): _____
Mean pulmonary artery pressure: _____
Pulmonary capillary wedge pressure: _____
Cardiac output: _____
Systemic arterial pressure (systolic/diastolic): _____
Mean systemic arterial pressure: _____

13. Sites for surgical insertion of a pulmonary artery catheter include all of the following *except*:
    A. The saphenous vein
    B. The internal jugular vein
    C. The subclavian vein
    D. The femoral vein

14. Pulmonary capillary wedge pressure is a reflection of all of the following *except*:
    A. Left atrial pressure
    B. Left ventricular end-diastolic pressure
    C. Left ventricular systolic pressure
    D. Left ventricular filling pressure

15. The dicrotic notch on the pulmonary artery waveform indicates:
    A. Aortic valve closure
    B. Tricuspid valve closure
    C. Mitral valve closure
    D. Pulmonic valve closure

16. Provide the formulas used to calculate the following hemodynamic variables.
Cardiac index (CI): _____
Stroke volume (SV): _____
Stroke index (SI): _____
Systemic vascular resistance (SVR): _____
Pulmonary vascular resistance (PVR): _____
Left ventricular stroke work index (LVSWI): _____
Right ventricular stroke work index (RVSWI): _____

17. High systemic vascular resistance is caused by:
    A. Arteriolar vessel constriction
    B. Low right atrial pressure
    C. Decreased blood volume
    D. Vasodilation

18. Right ventricular afterload is reflected by:
    A. Systemic vascular resistance
    B. Right atrial pressure
    C. Stroke volume
    D. Pulmonary vascular resistance

19. Of the following, the factor that would, by itself, cause PCWP to be disproportionate with left ventricular end-diastolic volume is:
    A. Mechanical ventilation with PEEP
    B. Hypovolemia
    C. Abnormal contractility
    D. Hypervolemia

III. Clinical Application of Hemodynamic Measurements

20. Write each of the following hemodynamic conditions in the appropriate quadrant of Forrester's hemodynamic subsets: normal hemodynamic state, acute left heart failure, hypervolemia, dehydration, septic shock, and myocardial infarction.

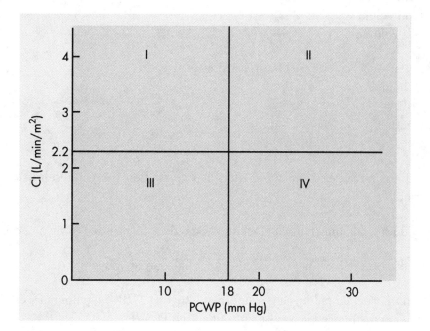

21. All of the following help reduce PCWP *except:*
    A. Diuretic drugs
    B. Inotropic drugs
    C. Vasoconstricting drugs
    D. Reduction of ventilation pressures

22. Vasodilator drugs improve hemodynamic status by:
    A. Decreasing ventricular ejection fraction
    B. Reducing resistance to ventricular ejection
    C. Increasing vascular tone
    D. Increasing myocardial oxygen consumption

23. Reduced myocardial contractility may be treated with all of the following *except:*
    A. Vasopressor drugs
    B. Inotropic drugs
    C. Vasodilator drugs
    D. IV fluids

▷ Putting It All Together

1. If cardiac contractility and valvular function are normal, an abnormally high PCWP is caused by:
   A. High left ventricular stroke volume
   B. Low systemic vascular resistance
   C. High blood volume
   D. Low blood volume

2. Oxygen delivery may be decreased by an extreme *increase* in:
   A. Stroke volume
   B. Contractility
   C. Cardiac output
   D. Heart rate

3. Bacterial endotoxins cause systemic vasodilation. Explain how this can result in abnormally high cardiac output.

4. In what way does a calcium channel blocking drug reduce myocardial oxygen consumption?

5. In what way does excessively high PEEP affect cardiac output and why?

6. Why does left ventricular failure cause abnormally high PCWP and pulmonary edema? In what situation could pulmonary edema exist without a high PCWP?

7. Noninvasive techniques for evaluating hemodynamic status include assessment of jugular venous distension (JVD). Of the pulmonary artery measurements CVP, MPAP, PCWP, and MAP, which may be elevated in the presence of JVD?

▷ Cases to Consider

1. You are caring for a patient in the intensive care unit who has a history of chronic obstructive pulmonary disease with chronic hypoxemia. A pulmonary artery catheter has been placed to monitor the patient's hemodynamic status. Current measurements from the catheter include: CVP = 12 mm Hg, PAP = 40/20 mm Hg, PCWP = 16 mm Hg, and cardiac output and LVSWI are below normal. The patient's body hydration appears appropriate, according to their baseline weight and laboratory studies. You recommend that a conservative dose of dopamine (see Table 17-5 in the text) be started for this patient. What benefits do you expect from this therapy? Why would this drug produce the expected benefits? What is a disadvantage of the drug for this type of patient?

2. Dopamine is administered to the patient in the case above. The hemodynamic measurements are now CVP = 5 mm Hg, PAP = 42/15 mm Hg, PCWP = 10 mm Hg, and cardiac output and LVSWI are within normal limits. Taking the patient's medical history into account, why is the systolic PAP value still abnormal? Comment on the effectiveness of the inotropic drug.

Section III
Integrated Function in Exercise

Chapter 18
Cardiopulmonary Response to Exercise in Health, Disease, and Aging

▷ Points to Remember

- Adenosine triphosphate (ATP) is the energy source for skeletal muscle activity; muscle stores of ATP must be continually regenerated.
- Aerobic synthesis of ATP uses oxygen supplied by the cardiovascular system until the demands of heavy exercise exceed oxygen delivery capacity.
- Anaerobic ATP synthesis occurs in the absence of oxygen and produces lactic acid.
- Maximal achievable heart rate limits cardiac output, imposing a normal limit to exercise intensity.
- A ventilatory limit to exercise exists when breathing reserve is exhausted but heart rate is less than maximal; a cardiovascular limit exists when cardiac output is insufficient but ventilatory reserve is not exhausted.
- Exercise tests identify appropriate heart rates and exercise intensities for individuals participating in cardiopulmonary rehabilitation.
- Even though ventilatory capacity is reduced in advancing age, ventilation does not normally limit exercise; increased stroke volume increases cardiac output appropriately in the healthy elderly adult.
- Age-related impairments to cardiac function are increased vascular resistance, reduced myocardial responsiveness to beta-adrenergic stimulation, and delayed ventricular relaxation.
- Increased left ventricular muscle mass and increased atrial contraction strength compensate for reduced cardiac function in healthy elderly adults.
- Maximal oxygen consumption in the elderly decreases because of reduced skeletal muscle mass.

▶ The Basics

I. Physiology of Exercise

1. The source of energy for skeletal muscle contraction is adenosine:
   A. Phosphate
   B. Monophosphate
   C. Diphosphate
   D. Triphosphate

2. ATP stores in skeletal muscle will sustain muscular activity for approximately:
   A. 1 minute
   B. 10 minutes
   C. 20 minutes
   D. 30 minutes

3. All of the following are formed or produced by aerobic metabolism *except*:
   A. O_2
   B. ATP
   C. CO_2
   D. H_2O

4. All of the following are involved in anaerobic glycolysis *except*:
   A. ATP
   B. Lactic acid
   C. Oxygen
   D. Pyruvic acid

5. At approximately what percentage of the body's maximal oxygen consumption ($\dot{V}O_{2max}$) does anaerobic threshold normally occur?
   A. 90%
   B. 80%
   C. 60%
   D. 50%

6. The respiratory quotient (RQ) for glucose is (greater than, less than) the RQ for fats.

7. A metabolic cart measures all of the following *except*:
   A. Exhaled CO_2 concentrations
   B. Electrocardiogram
   C. Tidal volume
   D. Minute ventilation

130 Integrated Function in Exercise

8. Number the following physiological changes in the order that they occur during exercise.
   _____ Exercise begins to intensify.
   _____ Oxygen consumption increases.
   _____ Pulse pressure rises significantly.
   _____ Contracting muscles consume increasing amounts of ATP.
   _____ Cardiac output increases.
   _____ Skeletal capillaries are recruited in working muscles.

9. The predicted maximal heart rate for a 65-year-old adult is:
   A. 120 beats/min
   B. 135 beats/min
   C. 155 beats/min
   D. 170 beats/min

10. During exercise, an unconditioned person and a conditioned athlete have the same:
    A. Maximal heart rate
    B. Stroke volume
    C. Maximum oxygen consumption
    D. Cardiac output

11. After anaerobic threshold is reached, continued exercise normally *accelerates* the rate of increase in all the following *except*:
    A. CO_2 production
    B. Oxygen consumption
    C. Minute ventilation
    D. Anaerobic glycolysis

12. After reaching anaerobic threshold in healthy individuals:
    A. Carbon dioxide production decreases
    B. Minute ventilation parallels oxygen consumption
    C. Oxygen consumption rate is constant
    D. Blood bicarbonate concentration begins to decrease

13. After the isocapnic buffering period, the minute ventilation slope normally becomes steeper because:
    A. Increased respiratory acidosis drives ventilation.
    B. Carbon dioxide production parallels minute ventilation.
    C. Metabolic acidosis provides additional ventilatory stimulus.
    D. The rate of oxygen consumption increases.

14. After anaerobic threshold is reached, all of the following arterial blood gas values normally decrease *except*:
    A. PaO_2
    B. $PaCO_2$
    C. pH
    D. HCO_3^-

15. If work done per minute remains constant and the body's energy cost per minute increases, work efficiency (increases, decreases).

16. If resting oxygen consumption equals twenty mets, oxygen consumption is equal to:
    A. 7 ml/min/kg
    B. 14 ml/min/kg
    C. 35 ml/min/kg
    D. 70 ml/min/kg

17. The normal primary limiting factor of exercise intensity is:
    A. Cardiac stroke volume
    B. Cardiac capacity
    C. Maximum attainable minute ventilation
    D. V_D/V_T

18. Normally, the heart rate reserve at maximum exercise is:
    A. 0
    B. 10 %
    C. 20 %
    D. 40 %

19. Decreases in all of the following are associated with decreases in oxygen pulse *except*:
    A. Stroke volume
    B. Arterial oxygen content
    C. Heart rate
    D. $C(a-\bar{v})O_2$

20. In what way does the response to exercise differ in physically fit versus physically unfit people of the same age performing the same work?
    A. The maximum heart rates are lower in physically unfit people.
    B. Oxygen consumption is lower for the same work in physically fit people.
    C. Oxygen delivery rate is higher in physically unfit people.
    D. Cardiac output is higher at a given heart rate in physically fit people.

II. Physiological Basis for Clinical Exercise Testing

21. On the graph below, draw a slope representing the heart rate/work rate relationship for an individual with poor stroke volume.

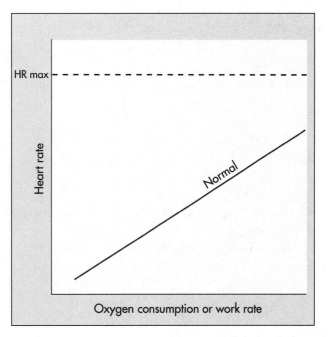

22. People with severe obstructive airways disease are limited during exercise because:
    A. They reach maximum heart rate before their ventilation limit
    B. They are unable to provide the minute ventilation required to do more work
    C. Their ability to eliminate CO_2 exceeds their ability to deliver O_2 to tissues
    D. They have above normal maximum voluntary ventilation

23. All of the following statements are true about the response to exercise of most patients with chronic obstructive pulmonary disease (COPD) *except*:
    A. They have an abnormally high resting minute ventilation.
    B. They are unable to reach anaerobic threshold.
    C. Their V_D/V_T increases during exercise.
    D. Their $\dot{V}/\dot{Q}$ mismatch may improve during exercise.

24. Compared to exercise test results of a patient with COPD, test results for a restrictive lung disease patient are typically different because restrictive lung disease has a(n):
    A. Lower breathing reserve
    B. Higher heart rate reserve at maximum exercise
    C. Breathing rate > 50/min at maximum exercise
    D. Inadequate $\dot{V}_E$ response to lactic acidosis

25. Exercise in endurance training should be high enough to produce a heart rate between:
    A. 80% and 100% of predicted maximum
    B. 80% and 90% of predicted maximum
    C. 60% and 80% of predicted maximum
    D. 60% and 70% of predicted maximum

III. Effects of Aging

26. Normal age-related changes in respiratory function include all of the following *except:*
    A. Decreased vital capacity
    B. Increased P(A-a)O_2
    C. Decreased maximum $\dot{V}O_2$
    D. Increased $PaCO_2$

27. Maximal oxygen consumption at peak exercise decreases with age mainly because of reductions in:
    A. Skeletal muscle mass
    B. Ventilation
    C. Cardiovascular function
    D. Oxygen delivery

28. Major age-related cardiovascular impairments normally include all of the following *except:*
    A. Increased vascular resistance
    B. Reduced response to beta-adrenergic stimulation
    C. Decreased cardiac output
    D. Hampered ventricular relaxation

▶ Putting It All Together

1. Why might a diet that is high in sugars and starches and low in fats pose a ventilatory problem for a chronically hypercapnic patient?

2. If the ability to hyperventilate is impaired by lung disease or ventilatory muscular abnormalities, does this affect oxygen debt, ATP synthesis, and blood pH? How?

3. In what way will the time required to reach maximum exercise be affected in an otherwise healthy individual with decreased ventricular ejection fraction? What will the heart rate reserve (HRR) be for this individual at maximum exercise? How does this individual's O_2 pulse compare to normal?

4. Why does an increased level of physical fitness decrease resting heart rate?

5. As work rate increases, oxygen consumption increases. Why does the rate of oxygen consumption *decline* during exercise in the presence of cardiac disease?

6. In what way does the HRR of a patient with COPD differ from normal HRR? Why?

▶ Cases to Consider

1. A 70-year-old male patient has completed an exercise test and you are to evaluate the test results. The patient's maximal heart rate was 150/min and, after reaching aerobic threshold, $\dot{V}CO_2/\dot{V}O_2$ increased modestly; breathing reserve was 30% of MVV; and minute ventilation and carbon dioxide elimination increased more rapidly than oxygen consumption. Comment on the test results compared to normal and state the heart rate reserve.

2. Results from a patient's exercise test yield the following information: ventilatory reserve at maximum exercise was greater than normal; heart rate rose more rapidly than $\dot{V}O_2$ (low O_2 pulse); maximum heart rate and anaerobic threshold were reached at a relatively low work rate; and the V_D/V_T ratio was high. Although the patient has no history of pulmonary disease, some of the test results are consistent with exercise in COPD. Which test results are consistent with those expected in COPD? Do the test results as a whole indicate pulmonary or cardiac exercise limitation?

Section IV
The Renal System

Chapter 19

Renal Regulation of Fluids, Electrolytes, and Acid-Base Balance

▶ Points To Remember

- The kidneys continually filter approximately 20% of the circulating blood plasma.
- The nephron is the functional unit of the kidney; its tubules reabsorb most of the filtrate back into the blood by active transport or passive diffusion.
- Autoregulatory feedback mechanisms in the kidneys maintain a constant glomerular filtration rate, even with large systemic blood pressure changes.
- Respiratory acid-base disturbances are compensated by titrating filtered HCO_3^- against secreted H^+ in the kidney.
- The body places a priority on sodium reabsorption, sometimes causing imbalances in potassium and hydrogen ions.
- Filtrate buffers are important in maintaining filtrate pH while excreting excess hydrogen ions.
- Renal failure is typified by impaired excretion of sodium, fixed acids, and end-products of protein breakdown; this results in fluid retention, metabolic acidosis, and high blood concentrations of urea and creatinine.
- Hyperventilation occurs in renal failure in an attempt to compensate for metabolic acidosis; this may cause ventilatory failure with pre-existing respiratory disease.

▷ The Basics

I. Functional Anatomy of the Kidney

1. On the illustration below, label the following structures: afferent arteriole, efferent arteriole, renal corpuscle, proximal convoluted tubule, loop of Henle, distal convoluted tubule, peritubular capillaries, vasa recta, and juxtaglomerular apparatus.

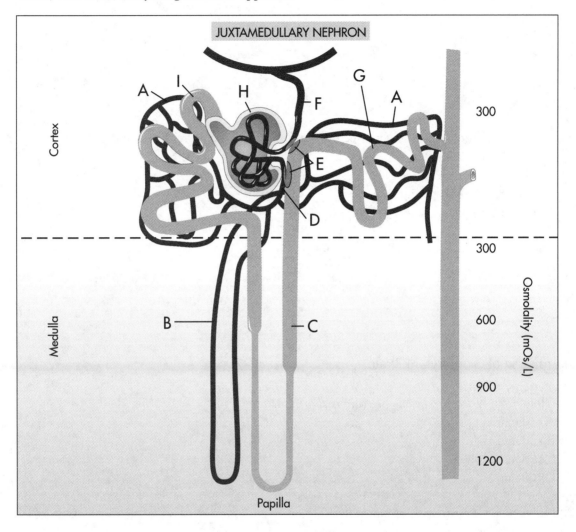

2. The basic functional unit of the kidney is called the:
   A. Glomerulus
   B. Nephron
   C. Cortex
   D. Convoluted tubule

3. The proximal and distal tubule are so named because they are positioned proximal and distal to the:
   A. Loop of Henle
   B. Bowman's capsule
   C. Collecting duct
   D. Renal corpuscle

4. The glomerulus is formed by a dense tuft of capillaries branching off of the:
   A. Efferent arteriole
   B. Peritubular arterioles
   C. Vasa recta
   D. Afferent arteriole

5. The percent of cardiac output flowing through the kidneys is:
   A. 100 %
   B. 60 %
   C. 40 %
   D. 20 %

6. Glomerular capillaries form a (high, low) pressure bed and peritubular capillaries form a (high, low) pressure bed.

7. Afferent and efferent arteriolar vasoconstriction occurs because renin is secreted by the:
   A. Renal corpuscle
   B. Glomerulus
   C. Juxtaglomerular apparatus
   D. Convoluted tubules

8. The nephron reabsorbs all of the following *except*:
   A. Water
   B. Urea
   C. Electrolytes
   D. Glucose

II. Formation of Glomerular Filtrate

9. Glomerular blood *hydrostatic* pressure is approximately:
   A. 10 mm Hg
   B. 30 mm Hg
   C. 50 mm Hg
   D. 60 mm Hg

10. Net *filtration* pressure is approximately:
    A. 10 mm Hg
    B. 30 mm Hg
    C. 50 mm Hg
    D. 60 mm Hg

11. Net filtration pressure is opposed by all of the following *except*:
    A. Capsular osmotic pressure
    B. Glomerular capillary pressure
    C. Glomerular osmotic pressure
    D. Capsular hydrostatic pressure

12. The process of filtration (increases, decreases) the osmotic pressure of efferent arteriole blood.

13. Total daily urine output is approximately:
    A. 700 ml
    B. 1000 ml
    C. 1500 ml
    D. 1800 ml

14. Non-threshold substances in glomerular filtrate include:
    A. Glucose
    B. Amino acids
    C. Phosphates
    D. Creatinine

15. Afferent arteriolar constriction (increases, decreases) glomerular filtration pressure, and efferent arteriolar constriction (increases, decreases) it.

III. Processing Glomerular Filtrate

16. Number the following structures in the order that filtrate flows through them.
    _____ Bowman's capsule
    _____ Distal convoluted tubule
    _____ Proximal convoluted tubule
    _____ Collecting duct
    _____ Loop of Henle

17. All of the following explain how high osmotic pressure is maintained in the medulla *except*:
    A. Cells of the ascending loop of Henle actively pump sodium ions from the medullary interstitial fluid into the filtrate.
    B. Sodium ions pumped out of the ascending loop of Henle immediately diffuse into the descending loop of Henle and the vasa recta.
    C. New sodium ions continually move from the proximal tubule into the loop of Henle.
    D. Sluggishly flowing blood in the vasa recta cannot effectively remove solutes from the medullary region.

18. When extracellular fluid volume (increases, decreases), aldosterone is secreted and the quantity of water in the urine (increases, decreases).

19. Antidiuretic hormone (ADH) is secreted by the:
    A. Pituitary gland
    B. Adrenal glands
    C. Atrial muscle fibers
    D. Macula densa

20. Urine volume is increased by increased secretion of:
    A. Renin
    B. Atrial natriuretic hormone
    C. Aldosterone
    D. Antidiuretic hormone

IV. Acid-Base and Electrolyte Regulation

21. The body places the highest priority on maintaining normal concentrations of:
    A. Potassium
    B. Sodium
    C. Chloride
    D. Bicarbonate

22. Primary active transport accounts for the majority of sodium ion reabsorption from tubular filtrate in all of the following *except* the:
    A. Proximal tubule
    B. Distal tubule
    C. Descending loop of Henle
    D. Ascending loop of Henle

23. In primary active transport, the ions that are normally transported from the blood into the tubular epithelial cells are the:
    A. Hydrogen ions
    B. Chloride ions
    C. Potassium ions
    D. Bicarbonate ions

24. In the process of secondary active secretion of potassium and hydrogen ions:
    A. Hydrogen is transported into the tubular cell.
    B. Sodium diffuses into the tubular cell.
    C. Potassium diffuses into the tubular cell.
    D. Chloride is transported into the tubular cell.

25. In most tubular segments, which ion is normally reabsorbed with sodium?
    A. Chloride
    B. Bicarbonate
    C. Potassium
    D. Hydrogen

26. Potassium diffuses into the filtrate through the luminal borders of tubular cells found only in the:
    A. Late distal tubule and cortical collecting duct
    B. Late proximal tubule and loop of Henle
    C. Loop of Henle and early distal tubule
    D. Proximal tubule and medullary collecting duct

27. Increased aldosterone secretion causes:
    A. Increased pumping of sodium into tubular cells
    B. Increased pumping of potassium out of tubular cells
    C. The sodium concentration in filtrate to rise
    D. The potassium concentration in filtrate to rise

28. If the number of bicarbonate ions and hydrogen ions passing into the tubular filtrate are equal to each other, there is:
    A. A net loss of base from the blood
    B. A net gain of acid in the blood
    C. A net gain of base in the blood
    D. No net loss of acid or base

29. Secondary active secretion of hydrogen ions occurs throughout the nephron *except* in the:
    A. Early proximal tubules
    B. Thin parts of the loop of Henle
    C. Late distal tubules
    D. Early distal tubules

30. When the kidney compensates for respiratory acidosis, the rate of hydrogen ion secretion is (greater than, less than) the rate of bicarbonate filtration into the tubules. For this to happen, the rate of carbon dioxide diffusion from the blood into tubule cells must be (greater than, less than) normal.

31. Hydrogen ions are transported in the urine by all of the following buffers *except*:
    A. Phosphate ions
    B. Ammonium ions
    C. Bicarbonate ions
    D. Ammonia molecules

32. Label the two illustrations below as either representing hyperkalemia or hypokalemia and acidemia or alkalemia.

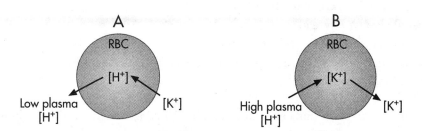

33. Causes of hypokalemia include all of the following *except*:
    A. Diarrhea
    B. Chronic hypercapnia
    C. Diuretic therapy
    D. Low dietary potassium intake

34. Deleterious effects of acidosis include all of the following *except*:
    A. Drowsiness
    B. Cardiac arrhythmias
    C. Hyperactive nervous system
    D. Coma

35. Glomerulonephritis, tubular necrosis, and blood transfusion reactions are all similar in that they are characterized by:
    A. Loss of normal filtrate flow in the tubules
    B. An abnormal immune reaction to microorganisms
    C. Renal ischemia
    D. Excess hemoglobin in the filtrate

36. Effects of chronic renal failure include all of the following *except*:
    A. General edema
    B. Metabolic acidosis
    C. Low blood concentrations of urea and creatinine
    D. High blood concentrations protein end-products

▶ Putting It All Together

1. Number the following events as they occur when the body becomes dehydrated.
   _____ Osmotic pressure changes, and water is reabsorbed from the filtrate.
   _____ Sodium is actively reabsorbed from the distal tubular filtrate.
   _____ Angiotensin II is formed.
   _____ Extracellular fluid volume falls below normal.
   _____ Adrenal glands secrete aldosterone.
   _____ Extracellular fluid volume is restored to normal.
   _____ Macula densa cells of the juxtaglomerular apparatus secrete renin.
   _____ Renal blood flow decreases.

2. A high dietary intake of sodium can result in an increased extracellular fluid volume. For each of the following substances, state whether the secretion rate is increased or decreased during high sodium intake.

Renin: _____
Aldosterone: _____
Atrial natriuretic hormone: _____
Antidiuretic hormone: _____

3. Increasing body fluid levels in a patient with congestive heart failure may present a pumping challenge that the failing heart is unable to meet. What is the mechanism by which the kidneys in a patient with congestive heart failure would actually *increase* water retention?

4. Of the following drugs, which one actually becomes the osmotic agent itself (instead of the body's own Na^+, Cl^-, or HCO_3^-) in the tubular filtrate:
   A. Acetazolamide
   B. Thiazide-type drugs
   C. Mannitol
   D. Furosemide

5. Why does infusion of potassium chloride correct elevated HCO_3^- in metabolic alkalosis?

6. Why does a loop diuretic, which increases sodium excretion, also lead to hypokalemia?

7. Explain why a chronically hypercapnic patient with COPD may tend to be hypochloremic and hypokalemic.

8. Explain why a potassium-depleting diuretic may cause alkalosis.

9. Why is it possible to cause cardiac arrhythmias in an alkalotic, hypokalemic patient by administering potassium chloride?

▶ A Case to Consider

You are caring for an elderly patient with COPD who was recently admitted to the respiratory unit of your medical center for an acute lung infection. The patient has chronic CO_2 retention and was acidotic at admission because arterial PCO_2 was elevated above baseline. Aggressive bronchodilator therapy has not kept pace with the patient's ventilatory status, as indicated by somewhat worsened bedside peak expiratory flow measurements and chest auscultation. The attending physician ordered laboratory studies 48 hours ago and again today. The results have been consistent with an acute infection coincidental with chronic hypercapnia and compensated respiratory acidosis (elevated white blood cell count and elevated total CO_2). Reviewing the laboratory test results, you notice that blood urea nitrogen (BUN) and creatinine (Cr) were elevated at admission time and have risen significantly since then. You contact the attending physician with the laboratory test results and a request for an arterial blood gas order. While making your request, you also inquire about the patient's wishes pertaining to life support, specifically, mechanical ventilation. Why is an arterial blood gas needed? What do you expect it to reveal? Why are you inquiring about mechanical ventilation?

Answer Key

Answer Key

Chapter 1: The Airways and Alveoli

The Basics
1. A. Middle meatus
   B. Inferior meatus
   C. Hard palate
   D. Lingual tonsil
   E. Epiglottis
   F. Vocal cord
   G. Thyroid cartilage
   H. Cricoid cartilage
   I. Trachea
   J. Superior meatus
   K. Opening of auditory tube
   L. Nasopharynx
   M. Soft palate
   N. Palantine tonsil
   O. Oropharynx
   P. Laryngopharynx
   Q. Esophagus
2. C
3. Nasopharynx, oropharynx, laryngopharynx
4. Nasopharynx, oropharynx
5. A
6. A. Thyroid cartilage
   B. Epiglottis
   C. Cricothyroid ligament
   D. Cricoid cartilage
   E. Corniculate cartilage
   F. Tracheal cartilage
   G. Vallecula
   H. Epiglottis
   I. True vocal cords
   J. False vocal cord
   K. Glottis (or trachea)
   L. Arytenoid cartilage
   M. Cuneiform cartilage
   N. Corniculate cartilage
7. Larynx
8. B
9. B
10. A
11. True vocal folds
12. D
13. Laryngospasm
14. Respiratory or gas exchange zone
15. 17 through 23
16. 1 through 16 (the conducting zone)
17. Carina, fifth
18. Left, right
19. Conducting airways: E
    Alveoli: C
    Clara cells: B
    Acinus: G
    Pores of Kohn: F
    Respiratory bronchioles: D
    Parenchyma: A
20. A. Mucous blanket
    B. Mucosa
    C. Epithelium
    D. Lamina propria
    E. Submucosa
    F. Adventitia
    G. Goblet cell
    H. Mucous gland
21. Goblet, submucosal mucous
22. Ciliated epithelial cells
23. Gel, sol
24. D
25. D
26. A
27. C

Putting It All Together
1. D
2. C
3. B
4. C
5. A
6. D
7. A

A Case to Consider
Abdominal movements indicate that the patient is making ventilatory effort. The fact that no signs of air movement are present suggests that an airway obstruction is present. Initial suspicions would certainly include soft tissue (e.g., the tongue) occlusion of the upper airway. An upper airway occlusion results in the loss of air exchange while ventilatory effort continues.

Chapter 2: The Lungs and Chest Wall

The Basics

1. A. Thyroid cartilage
   B. Right heart border
   C. Right diaphragm border
   D. Liver
   E. Sternum
   F. Stomach
   G. Left diaphragm border
   H. Left heart border
   I. Cardiac notch
   J. Clavicle
   K. Lung apex
   L. Trachea
2. B
3. D
4. Heart, liver
5. A. Thyroid cartilage
   B. Cricoid cartilage
   C. Larynx
   D. Trachea
   E. Right bronchus
   F. Parietal pleura
   G. Visceral pleura
   H. Diaphragm
   I. Pleural space
   J. Mediastinum
   K. Left bronchus
   L. Aorta
6. Connects visceral pleura with diaphragm: D
   Left lung portion overlapping heart: G
   Attached to inner chest wall surface: H
   Between visceral and parietal membranes: A
   Diaphragm meets chest wall: B
   Result of inflamed pleural space: F
   Tube in pleural cavity: C
   Air in pleural space: E
7. A
8. C
9. D
10. A
11. Higher
12. B
13. Chest wall muscles: S
    Lung: A
    Airway smooth muscle: A
    Voluntary motor control: S
    Phrenic nerves: S
    Diaphragm: S
    Vagus nerve: A
    Intercostal nerves: S
14. Parasympathetic, sympathetic, NANC, NANC
15. D
16. A
17. D
18. B
19. Vagus: B
    Deep inspiration: E
    Slowly adapting receptors: F
    Rapidly adapting receptors: A
    Cough reflex: G
    J-receptors: D
    C-fiber receptors: C
20. Abdominal muscles contract forcefully: 4
    Diaphragm contracts: 1
    Glottis opens suddenly: 5
    Larynx muscles close the glottis: 3
    Inspiratory pause: 2
21. Pump handle, bucket handle
22. C
23. C
24. C
25. B
26. Floating: C
    Vertebrosternal: F
    Vertebrochondral: D
    Costal groove: E
    Manubrium: H
    Body: A
    Xiphoid: G
    Angle of Louis: B

Putting It All Together

1. C
2. D
3. D
4. A
5. A
6. B
7. D
8. B
9. C

Cases to Consider

1. The patient's signs are all consistent with chronic obstructive pulmonary disease (COPD). Elevated shoulders and tensing neck muscles show that accessory muscle use is occurring, indicating increased work of breathing. Increased work of breathing and a flattened diaphragm secondary to hyperinflation indicate that chronic airway obstruction is present.

2. Wheezing indicates that airway obstruction exists. Since the wheezing does not clear when secretions are cleared from the airways, airway obstruction is probably the result of bronchoconstriction. The inhaled acetylcysteine caused airway irritation, smooth muscle spasming, and airway narrowing. A bronchodilator type drug must be used to reverse bronchoconstriction and open airways to their normal diameters.

Chapter 3: The Mechanics of Ventilation

The Basics

1. Recoil force: D
   Contributes most to lung elasticity: F
   Mouth pressure during spontaneous breathing: A
   Alveolar pressure: B
   Pressure between chest wall and lung: I
   Difference between two pressures: C
   No flow of air: J
   Alveolar minus atmospheric pressure: G
   Alveolar minus pleural pressure: E
   Intrapleural minus atmospheric pressure: H
2. A. Airway opening (mouth) pressure
   B. Alveolar (intrapulmonary) pressure
   C. Intrapleural pressure
   D. Body surface pressure
   E. Transrespiratory pressure
   F. Transpulmonary pressure
   G. Transthoracic pressure
3. B
4. B
5. A
6. Capacity: B
   Volume: H
   Total lung capacity: I
   Residual volume: F
   Vital capacity: A
   Inspiratory capacity: C
   Expiratory reserve volume: E
   Functional residual capacity: G
   Tidal volume: D
7. C
8. C
9. B
10. C
11. D
12. C
13. B
14. D
15. Increases
16. C
17. C
18. A
19. C
20. B
21. D
22. C
23. Driving pressure: B
    Viscosity: A
    Laminar flow: F
    Turbulent flow: C
    Poiseuille's law: D
    Transitional flow: E
24. B
25. D
26. C
27. C
28. Total compliance is decreased: C
    Total compliance is increased: A
    Residual volume percent of total lung capacity is increased: A
    Lung compliance is normal: B
    Lung compliance is increased: A
    Lung compliance is consistent with chronic obstructive pulmonary disease: A
    Lung compliance is consistent with fibrotic lung disease: C
    High lung recoil force is present: C
    Low lung recoil force is present: A
29. A
30. D
31. B
32. C
33. B
34. C
35. A

Putting It All Together

1. Apical regions exist in a distended state and tend to have higher alveolar pressures. They are less compliant and therefore more susceptible to insults to the parenchyma (disease, high pressure, increased ventilatory demand).
2. D
3. C, D, F, H
4. B
5. A
6. C
7. A
8. D
9. B
10. C

Cases to Consider

1. Since the patient's lungs are clear and seem to be free of unwanted secretions, the increased difference between peak and plateau pressures is probably not due to poor conducting airway patency. However, in this scenario, the involuntary muscle contractions can easily cause biting of the endotracheal tube, yielding high peak inspiratory pressures and normal plateau pressures.
2. Ventilatory muscle strength and the ability to maintain adequate ventilation are threatened in this patient. As the primary muscle of inspiration, the diaphragm is a focus of concern. Maximum inspiratory pressure is a measure of ventilatory muscle strength and assists in evaluating ability to ventilate. Inspiratory capacity or vital capacity are volume measurements that also indicate ventilatory strength.
3. The physicians probably suspect the damage to the patient's airway includes alveolar epithelial damage, reducing natural pulmonary surfactant levels. Since surfactant reduces alveolar surface tension, it directly affects the inspiratory pressure required to open alveoli. Low surfactant levels would cause significant alveolar collapse and concomitant high work of breathing.

Chapter 4: Ventilation

The Basics

1. Nitrogen: C
   Oxygen: F
   Carbon dioxide: A
   Barometric pressure: B
   Dalton's law: E
   Water vapor: D
2. D
3. D
4. B
5. Tidal volume, breathing frequency
6. A
7. C
8. B
9. B
10. A. Patient A: 4.5 L   Patient B: 5.6 L
    B. Patient A: 1.5 L   Patient B: 2.4 L
    C. Patient A: 3.0 L   Patient B: 3.2 L
    D. Patient A: 67%   Patient B: 57%
    E. Patient A: 33%   Patient B: 43%
11. B
12. A
13. D
14. B
15. C

Putting It All Together

1. A
2. C
3. Patient A. Patient A has a larger alveolar ventilation percent and is receiving similar benefit from alveolar minute ventilation from a smaller minute ventilation.
4. Greater, smaller, greater, smaller, minute ventilation
5. Estimated anatomical deadspace: 1 ml/pound body weight = 200 ml
   Minute ventilation: 600 ml tidal volume × 15 breathing frequency = 9000 ml or 9.0 L
   Alveolar ventilation: 9000 ml − (15 × 200 ml)
     = 9000 ml − 3000 ml = 6000 ml or 6.0 L
   Deadspace/tidal volume ratio: 200/600 = 0.33 or 33% or 1/3
   Alveolar ventilation required to reduce arterial carbon dioxide to 40 mm Hg:
     45 × 6.0 = 40 × (new alveolar ventilation)
     270 = 40 × (new alveolar ventilation)
     270/40 = new alveolar ventilation
     6.75 L = new alveolar ventilation
   Minute ventilation needed for new alveolar ventilation:
   If deadspace/tidal volume ratio = 0.33, then alveolar/minute ventilation ratio = 0.67
     0.67 = 6.75/(new minute ventilation)
     0.67 × (new minute ventilation) = 6.75
     new minute ventilation = 10.1 L/min

6. B
7. B
8. B

Cases to Consider
1. The additional tubing will add 100 ml of deadspace to existing endotracheal tube and conducting airways deadspace. Since the patient receives only mechanical constant volume breaths, this additional deadspace will be subtracted from the volume of fresh gas reaching the alveoli. Since alveolar ventilation (and metabolic rate) determines alveolar and arterial carbon dioxide levels, alveolar ventilation will be effectively reduced by the additional deadspace. Arterial carbon dioxide will rise as alveolar ventilation falls. Without additional data, only an arterial blood sample could determine if hypercapnia actually occurs. The request could be honored if the tidal volume were increased by the volume of the additional deadspace tubing. This would negate the adverse effects of additional deadspace ventilation on alveolar ventilation.
2. Emphysema impairs the ability to normalize arterial carbon dioxide levels because of alveolar-capillary membrane destruction and reduced alveolar ventilation. The patient, with compromised alveolar ventilation, must increase her ventilatory effort to accommodate any increased demand to eliminate carbon dioxide. The physician noted, in the absence of other predisposing factors (acute pulmonary infection or significant worsening of premature airway collapse) that arterial carbon dioxide was at the patient's normal baseline, despite increased ventilation. The presence of normal baseline PCO_2 in spite of abnormal baseline ventilation demonstrates a physiologic response to increased CO_2 production. The patient interview revealed the source of increased CO_2 production and with it the dietary solution to a ventilation problem.
3. The patient originally presented with an arterial carbon dioxide concentration of 34 mm Hg and a breathing rate of 38, indicating an inefficient ventilatory response to low PaO_2. After the first 30 minutes, the patient's PaO_2 is still abnormally low and arterial carbon dioxide concentration has risen dramatically, reflecting poor ventilation secondary to patient fatigue and impending ventilatory failure. Mechanical ventilation is indicated to provide ventilatory support, correct hypoventilation, and reduce hypercapnia.

Chapter 5: Pulmonary Function Measurements

The Basics
1. B
2. C
3.

Degree of impairment	% Predicted
Normal	80% to 120%
Mild	65% to 79%
Moderate	50% to 64%
Severe	35% to 49%
Very severe	Less than 35%

(From Scanlan CL, Spearman CB, Sheldon RL: *Egan's fundamentals of respiratory care*, ed 6, St Louis, 1995, Mosby.)

4. D
5. A
6. B
7. C
8. D
9. D
10. A
11. A. IC: 3600 ml
    B. FRC: 2400 ml
    C. IRV: 3100 ml
    D. TV: 500 ml
    E. ERV: 1200 ml
    F. RV: 1200 ml
    G. VC: 4800 ml
    H. TLC: 6000 ml
12. B
13. C
14. B
15. D
16. A
17. Independent
18. D
19. D
20. A. Obstructive
    B. Restrictive
    C. Normal
21. D
22. A
23. B
24. C

25.

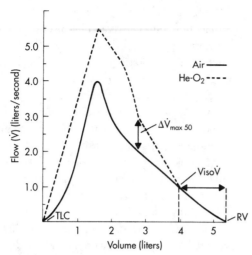

(From Ruppel G: *Manual of pulmonary function testing*, ed 6, St Louis, 1994, Mosby.)

Putting It All Together
1. C
2. A
3. A
4. Because FVC is a forced expiratory maneuver, early airway compression occurs in obstructive disease processes. Early airway compression results in a subnormal FVC value, similar to that in restrictive processes. FEV_1 is reduced in airway obstruction because of high expiratory airway resistance. In restrictive disease, FEV_1 is reduced because its reference volume, FVC, is also reduced. $FEV_1\%$ is normal or elevated in restrictive disease because both the numerator and denominator in the FEV_1/FVC ratio are proportionately reduced. FEV_1 is disproportionately lower than FVC in obstructive disease, resulting in a reduced FEV_1/FVC ratio.
5. C

Chapter 6: Pulmonary Blood Flow

The Basics
1. Systemic arterioles: 9
   Left ventricle: 7
   Systemic arteries: 8
   Right atrium: 1
   Pulmonary artery: 3
   Pulmonary veins: 5
   Pulmonic valve: 2
   Mitral valve: 6
   Pulmonary capillaries: 4
2. C
3. C
4. Balloon: E, F, G
   Thermistor: B

6. A
7. B
8. D

Cases to Consider
1. Obstructive lung disease is present in this patient. The values for FVC, FEV_1, and $FEV_1\%$ are beyond 20% deviation from average normal values. $FEV_1\%$ value reflects an obstructive disease process. All spirometric values are consistent with a significant reduction in expiratory flowrates. A diagnosis of emphysema for this patient is supported by a significant smoking history and documented lack of response to bronchodilator therapy. Additional testing by helium dilution or nitrogen washout alone would not conclusively support an obstructive diagnosis because these tests do not measure trapped gas. Body plethysmography will reflect any increases in FRC (consistent with emphysema) in this patient—even in the presence of air trapping.
2. The portion of the patient's history given here is consistent with a restrictive disease process. Pulmonary sarcoidosis and (grossly) normal peak flows point to reduced lung volumes and normal airways. Compared to helium dilution, nitrogen washout, or plethysmography, an FVC test is relatively simple and inexpensive to administer. An FVC maneuver will provide FVC, FEV_1 and $FEV_1\%$ values through which a restrictive diagnosis can possibly be made. For example, a low FVC with a normal $FEV_1\%$ confirms a restrictive diagnosis. The major indicator of obstructive disease in this instance would be a low $FEV_1\%$, accompanied by a low FEV_1. In addition, $FEF_{25\%-75\%}$ will be low in the presence of small airways disease.

Proximal lumen: B, C
Distal lumen: A, D, E, G
5. D
6. B
7. C
8. A
9. Pulmonary capillary recruitment: P
   Alveolar pressure: P
   Left ventricular failure: P
   Endogenous nitric oxide: A
   Low P_AO_2: A
   Arterial pH less than 7.30: A
   Systemic blood loss: P
10. C

Answer Key 151

11. A
12. A
13. D
14. B
15. A
16. B
17. D
18. C
19. A
20. C
21. A
22. A
23. C

Putting It All Together
1. D
2. D
3. B
4. Decreased blood volume decreases cardiac output, leading to collapse of pulmonary capillaries, low PAP, and increased PVR. Administering fluids in this situation promotes increased blood volume and cardiac output. Increased cardiac output improves vascular pressures, which, in turn, recruit and distend pulmonary vasculature, lowering PVR.
5. C
6. C
7. B
8. D
9. C

Cases to Consider
1. The hemodynamic values are indicative of left ventricular failure. The high PCWP (LVEDP) together with low cardiac output reflects poor left ventricular contractility. Decreased left ventricular contractility is also reflected in a low systemic blood pressure. High PAP is consistent with either high PVR or left ventricular failure. In this case, the PVR is low normal and the PAP-PCWP difference is normal, indicating a cardiac cause for elevated PAP. The low normal PVR is a by-product of pulmonary vascular distention and recruitment caused by increased PAP. Through increased hydrostatic pressure, high PCWP causes engorgement of pulmonary capillaries and, in this case, pulmonary edema. Secondary to pulmonary edema, alveolar collapse occurred and produced hypoxemia, increased work of breathing, and, eventually, respiratory distress. Mechanical ventilation was required to provide ventilatory support and restore adequate tissue oxygenation.
2. The mucous plug was the direct cause of increased work of breathing and decreased breath sounds. Indirectly, the compromised airway resulted in hypoxemia, which stimulated increased breathing frequency and hypoxic pulmonary vasoconstriction. HPV causes increased PVR and PAP. Removing the mucous plug decreased work of breathing, reduced breathing frequency, and restored previously compromised alveolar ventilation. Improved alveolar ventilation relieved alveolar hypoxia and, hence, removed the stimulus for HPV. As HPV subsided, PVR and PAP decreased as well. Increased alveolar oxygenation was also reflected in improved arterial oxygenation.
3. Normal PCWP indicates that left ventricular function is appropriate, so the cause of high PAP and CVP exists elsewhere. Chronic hypoxemia, secondary to alveolar-capillary membrane destruction from emphysema, has initiated a sequence of adverse hemodynamic events for this patient. Persistent hypoxic vasoconstriction has increased PAP. Long-term pumping against high PAP has produced right ventricular hypertrophy. Now, upstream pressures have elevated as well and CVP is above normal.

Chapter 7: Gas Diffusion

The Basics
1. A. Top arrow: oxygen; bottom arrow: carbon dioxide
   B. $P_{A_{O_2}} = 100$ mm Hg; $P_{A_{CO_2}} = 40$ mm Hg
   C. Oxygen diffusion = 250 ml/min; carbon dioxide diffusion = 200 ml/min
2. A
3. B
4. 0 mm Hg: G
   6 mm Hg: A
   40 mm Hg: C
   47 mm Hg: H
   46 mm Hg: D
   60 mm Hg: F
   100 mm Hg: E
   160 mm Hg: B
5. B
6. C
7. C
8. B
9. D
10. B
11. A
12. C

13. C
14. A. Diffusion limitation
    B. Perfusion limitation
15. A
16. B
17. Anemia: U
    Interstitial fibrosis: P
    Engorged capillaries: P
    High carbon monoxide blood levels: U
    Destruction of alveolar-capillary bed: S
    Regional atelectasis: M
    Pulmonary embolus: S
    Lobar pneumonia: M
18. D

Putting It All Together
1. B
2. D
3. A
4. B
5. B
6. Compression of a pulmonary artery can potentially reduce pulmonary blood flow and, therefore, capillary blood flow. The test gas must be one with a rate of diffusion that is determined by pulmonary capillary blood flow. Nitrous oxide transfer across the a-c membrane is perfusion limited. Therefore, reduced nitrous oxide uptake reflects a reduction in capillary blood flow.
7. D
8. A

Cases to Consider
1. The patient's diffusion capacity is probably reduced because of ventilation-perfusion mismatch secondary to atelectasis. This is indicated by low inspiratory lung volumes and auscultated inspiratory crackles. Poor pain control has resulted in general immobility and an inability to maintain normal lung expansion. Adequate pain control will allow an appropriate level of ambulation, improve lung volumes, resolve ventilation-perfusion mismatch, and increase diffusion capacity.
2. Spirometry has shown that a restrictive disease process is present. Given the worker's occupational history and current breath sounds, the restrictive process is probably the result of interstitial fibrosis. The pulmonary stress test has identified that oxygen transfer does not keep pace with oxygen consumption during exercise. A D_LCO will likely reflect increased diffusion path distance secondary to interstitial fibrosis, typified by normal oxygenation at rest and suboptimal oxygenation during exercise.

Chapter 8: Oxygen Equilibrium and Transport

The Basics
1. A
2. C
3. D
4. 20 ml oxygen/dl × 10 = 200 ml oxygen/L
   4 L/min × 200 ml oxygen/L = 800 ml oxygen/min
5. Yes, resting tissue oxygen uptake is about 250 ml/min.
6. B
7. A
8. B
9. D
10. $CaO_2 = (Hb \times 1.34 \times SO_2) + (PO_2 \times 0.003)$
11. B
12. SO_2, PO_2
13. B
14. C
15. D
16. Beginning at a PO_2 of 20 mm Hg, a 40 mm Hg increase produces 12 ml/dl increase in oxygen content. A 40 mm Hg increase from 60 to 100 mm Hg increases the oxygen content less than 2 ml/dl.
17. Right shift: increased PCO_2, decreased pH, increased temperature, increased 2,3-DPG levels
    Left shift: decreased PCO_2, increased pH, decreased temperature, decreased 2,3-DPG levels
18. Increases, increasing, increases, decreased
19. Volume of O_2 for each g Hb: F
    Total arterial oxygen content: A
    Total venous oxygen content: E
    Arterial-venous oxygen content difference: B
    Oxygen extraction ratio: C
    Dissolved arterial oxygen content: D
    Dissolved venous oxygen content: G
20. $CaO_2 = (12 \times 1.34 \times 0.95) + (95 \times 0.003)$
    $CaO_2 = (15.3 \text{ ml/dl}) + (0.3 \text{ ml/dl})$
    $CaO_2 = 15.6 \text{ ml/dl}$

21. $CaO_2 = (14 \times 1.34 \times .9) + (65 \times 0.003)$
    $CaO_2 = (16.9 \text{ ml/dl}) + (0.2 \text{ ml/dl})$
    $CaO_2 = 17.1 \text{ ml/dl}$
    $CvO_2 = (14 \times 1.34 \times .68) + (40 \times 0.003)$
    $CvO_2 = (12.8 \text{ ml/dl}) + (0.1 \text{ ml/dl})$
    $CvO_2 = 12.9 \text{ ml/dl}$
    $O_2 \text{ ER} = (17.1 \text{ ml/dl} - 12.9 \text{ ml/dl})/17.1 \text{ ml/dl}$
    $O_2 \text{ ER} = 4.2 \text{ ml/dl}/17.1 \text{ ml/dl}$
    $O_2 \text{ ER} = 0.25 \text{ or } 25\%$

22. A
23. B
24. A
25. B
26. B
27. C

Putting It All Together

1. Cyanosis usually occurs whenever the volume of desaturated hemoglobin concentration is at least 5 g/dl, whether in the presence of polycythemia (elevated hemoglobin concentration), anemia (low hemoglobin concentration), or normal hemoglobin concentration.

2. Each mm Hg of oxygen partial pressure yields a dissolved oxygen volume of 0.003 ml/dl. A PO_2 of 100 mm Hg equals 0.3 ml/dl dissolved oxygen content, which is only 1.5% of normal total oxygen content. A PO_2 of 333 mm Hg is required under otherwise normal conditions to provide even 1 ml/dl or 5% of total oxygen content. However, dissolved oxygen content may be clinically significant in situations where oxyhemoglobin content is severely decreased (abnormal hemoglobin, very low hemoglobin, high oxygen extraction ratio).

3. Increasing the SaO_2 to 100% increases the oxyhemoglobin content by 0.6 ml/dl:
   $8.0 \text{ g/dl} \times 1.34 \text{ ml/g Hb} \times 0.94 = 10.1 \text{ ml/dl}$
   $8.0 \text{ g/dl} \times 1.34 \text{ ml/g} \times 1.00 = 10.7 \text{ ml/dl}$
   $10.7 - 10.1 = 0.6 \text{ ml/dl}$ increase in oxyhemoglobin content

   An additional 2 g/dl Hb increases oxyhemoglobin content by 2.5 ml/dl:
   $10 \text{ g/dl} \times 1.34 \text{ ml/dl} \times 0.94 = 12.6 \text{ ml/dl}$
   $12.6 - 10.1 = 2.5 \text{ ml/dl}$ increase in oxyhemoglobin content

   Therefore, providing additional oxygen carrying capacity in this case results in a greater increase in oxygen content than simply increasing the saturation of existing hemoglobin concentration.

4. In either scenario, oxygen content will increase by 10%:
   $CaO_2 = \text{Hb} \times 1.34 \times 0.9$
   $CaO_2 = \text{Hb} \times 1.34 \times 0.99$
   $CaO_2 = \text{Hb}(1.21)$
   $CaO_2 = \text{Hb}(1.33)$
   $\text{Hb}(1.33) - \text{Hb}(1.21)/\text{Hb}(1.21) = 0.1 \text{ or } 10\%$
   $CaO_2 = 10 \times 1.34 \times SaO_2$
   $CaO_2 = 11 \times 1.34 \times SaO_2$
   $CaO_2 = 13.4(SaO_2)$
   $CaO_2 = 14.74(SaO_2)$
   $14.74(SaO_2) - 13.4(SaO_2)/13.4(SaO_2) = 0.1 \text{ or } 10\%$

5. In smoke inhalation patients, carbon monoxide crosses the alveolar-capillary membrane and competes with oxygen for hemoglobin binding sites. The portable pulse oximeter detects only the presence of deoxyhemoglobin and oxyhemoglobin, reflecting an erroneously high SaO_2. The CO oximeter, differentiating between variant forms of hemoglobin, provides an accurate SaO_2, which, in this case, is significantly below normal. Results from the CO oximeter for this patient will also reveal the presence of carboxyhemoglobin in the blood. Carboxyhemoglobin has a bright red color and is responsible for the patient's "rosy" color. Even though the patient may actually be hypoxic, cyanosis does not appear.

6. D

7. Right. Increased tissue metabolism, indicated here by increased tissue oxygen demand, increases CO_2 production and secondarily lowers pH, shifting the curve to the right. The right shift is also enhanced by elevated body temperature (fever), which in this case is caused by the infectious process and immune response.

Cases to Consider

1. The above normal $PaCO_2$ (a reflection of high P_ACO_2) indicates that hypoventilation exists. Above normal $PaCO_2$ and low pH will cause a right shift in the oxyhemoglobin curve. The right-shifted curve results in decreased hemoglobin affinity for oxygen and subsequently, increased oxygen unloading. This is evidenced by a PaO_2 that is abnormally high for an oxygen saturation of 88%. Since a PaO_2 of 60 normally yields an SaO_2 of 90%, a PaO_2 of 75 normally yields an SaO_2 greater than 90%. A reduction in the level of pain medications may correct hypoventilation by removing ventilatory depression. Positive pressure ventilatory support will also improve alveolar ventilation, if pain medication reduction is not possible.

2. The oxyhemoglobin curve shifted to the left, evidenced by an SaO_2 of 98% with an associated PO_2 of 70. An SaO_2 of 98% is normally associated with a PO_2 of about 100. In this situation, the curve shift is probably the result of administering stored blood, which has decreased 2,3 DPG levels, causing a left shift in the oxyhemoglobin curve. Since PCO_2 and pH are now within normal limits, they do not affect the position of the curve. Initially, hemoglobin oxygen content was 7.2 ml/dl (6.0 g/dl × 1.34 ml O_2/g × 0.90 = 7.2 ml/dl). Now, hemoglobin oxygen content is 15.8 ml/dl (12.0 g/dl × 1.34 ml O_2/g × 0.98 = 15.8 ml/dl). Doubling the patient's hemoglobin volume exactly doubles the hemoglobin oxygen content, if SaO_2 remains the same. In this case, oxygen content more than doubled because SaO_2 increased as well.

3. The oxyhemoglobin curve is left-shifted as evidenced by an abnormally high SaO_2 for the associated PaO_2 (with a PaO_2 of 65, SaO_2 should be slightly above 90%). With the information given, the left shift of the oxyhemoglobin curve is due, at least in part, to low body temperature. Warming the patient will improve hemoglobin oxygen release (moving the curve to the right), raise the volume of dissolved oxygen (and PaO_2), and increase the oxygen tension gradient between the blood and tissues, enhancing tissue oxygen uptake. Drawing a venous sample will allow you to calculate an arterial-venous oxygen content difference and accurately assess oxygen extraction ratio. Calculated oxygen transport for this patient is:

CaO_2 = (13.0 g/dl × 1.34 ml/g × 0.98) + (65 mm Hg × 0.003 ml/mm Hg)
CaO_2 = 17.07 + 0.20
CaO_2 = 17.27 ml/dl

O_2 DEL = (17.27 ml/dl × 10 dl/L) × 4.8 L/min
O_2 DEL = 172.7 ml/L × 4.8 L/min
O_2 DEL = 829 ml/min

If you find tissue oxygen consumption is normal (250 ml/min), the oxygen extraction ratio then is 30% (above normal) but oxygen delivery is still adequate.

4. $C\bar{v}O_2$ = (13.0 g/dl × 1.34 ml/g × 0.68) + (38 mm Hg × 0.003 ml/mm Hg)
$C\bar{v}O_2$ = 11.85 + 0.114
$C\bar{v}O_2$ = 11.96

$\dot{V}O_2$ = [C(a-v)O_2 × 10] × Q
$\dot{V}O_2$ = [(17.27 − 11.96) × 10] × 4.8
$\dot{V}O_2$ = (5.31 × 10) × 4.8
$\dot{V}O_2$ = 254.88 ml O_2/min

O_2 ER = C(a-$\bar{v}$) O_2/CaO_2
O_2 ER = 5.31 / 17.27
O_2 ER = 0.31 or 31%

Chapter 9: Carbon Dioxide Equilibrium and Transport

The Basics
1. B
2. D
3. $H_2O + CO_2 \longrightarrow H_2CO_3 \longrightarrow HCO_3^- + H^+$
4. A
5. A. 200 ml/min
   B. 40 mm Hg
   C. 200 ml/min
   D. 40 mm Hg
6. Alveolar PCO_2 does not decrease during hypoventilation.
   Plasma PCO_2 increases: 2
   Alveolar PCO_2 increases: 1
   Dissolved CO_2 increases: 3
   H_2CO_3 concentration increases: 4
   H_2CO_3 concentration does not decrease during hypoventilation.
7. The illustration on the left is hypoventilation; right-shifted; 1:1.
   The illustration on the right is hyperventilation; left-shifted; 1:1.
8. C
9. A
10. A
11. C
12. D
13. C
14. C
15. A

Putting It All Together
1. Increases, increases, decreases
2. Increased alveolar carbon dioxide partial pressure: F
   Decreased plasma carbon dioxide partial pressure: T
   Decreased carbonic acid: T
   Increased hydrogen ion concentration: F
   Right-shifted hydration reaction: F
   Left-shifted hydration equilibrium point: T
   Normal carbon dioxide tissue production/alveolar elimination ratio: T
3. C
4. Decreased

Cases to Consider
1. The abnormally low pH indicates an abnormally high H^+ ion concentration. The H^+ ion concentration here is the result of lactic acidosis, secondary to anaerobic tissue metabolism. Although mechanical ventilation will not directly eliminate lactic acid, it can be used to correct the H^+ ion concentration and, consequently, the pH level. Although the PCO_2 is within the normal physiologic range of 35 to 40 mm Hg, additional CO_2 elimination will improve blood pH. Hyperventilating the patient (by judiciously increasing tidal volume, breathing frequency, or both) will decrease alveolar and arterial CO_2. When CO_2 concentration is decreased, the hydration reaction is shifted to the left and the H^+ ion concentration is reduced, thereby raising pH toward normal.

2. The blood gas results indicate that a left shift in the hydration reaction has indeed occurred and that the patient is no longer acidotic. In fact, with a pH of 7.5, the H^+ ion concentration is below normal and an alkalemic state now exists. The original adjustments to the breathing frequency have resulted in excessive CO_2 elimination in relation to nonrespiratory H^+ ion production (increased alveolar ventilation may now be too high for the amount of lactic acid present). The breathing frequency may now be reduced. This reduction will decrease alveolar ventilation, allowing the CO_2 and blood H^+ ion concentration to rise, thereby decreasing pH.

Chapter 10: Acid-Base Regulation

The Basics
1. C
2. B
3. C
4. D
5. B
6. B
7. C
8. D
9. A
10. A
11. C
12. Decrease
13. Increase
14. D
15. Nonbicarbonate
16. B
17. B
18. pH = 6.1 + log[24/(45 × 0.03)]
    pH = 6.1 + log[24/1.35]
    pH = 6.1 + log[17.78]
    pH = 6.1 + 1.25
    pH = 7.35
19. $[HCO_3^-]$ = antilog(pH − 6.1) × ($PaCO_2$ × 0.03)
    $[HCO_3^-]$ = antilog(7.29 − 6.1) × (30 × 0.03)
    $[HCO_3^-]$ = antilog(1.19) × 0.9
    $[HCO_3^-]$ = 15.49 × 0.9
    $[HCO_3^-]$ = 13.9 mEq/L
20. $PaCO_2$ = $[HCO_3^-]$ / (antilog[pH − 6.1] × 0.03)
    $PaCO_2$ = 24 / (antilog[7.52 − 6.1] × 0.03)
    $PaCO_2$ = 24 / (antilog(1.42) × 0.03)
    $PaCO_2$ = 24 / (26.3 × 0.03)
    $PaCO_2$ = 24 / 0.789
    $PaCO_2$ = 30.4 mm Hg
21. C
22. C
23. A
24. D
25. B
26. D
27. C

28.

Acid-Base Disorder	Primary Defect	Compensatory Response
Respiratory acidosis	$\left[\dfrac{\rightarrow HCO_3^-}{\uparrow PaCO_2}\right] = \downarrow pH$	$\left[\dfrac{\uparrow HCO_3^-}{\uparrow PaCO_2}\right] = \rightarrow pH$
Respiratory alkalosis	$\left[\dfrac{\rightarrow HCO_3^-}{\downarrow PaCO_2}\right] = \uparrow pH$	$\left[\dfrac{\downarrow HCO_3^-}{\downarrow PaCO_2}\right] = \rightarrow pH$
Metabolic acidosis	$\left[\dfrac{\downarrow HCO_3^-}{\rightarrow PaCO_2}\right] = \downarrow pH$	$\left[\dfrac{\downarrow HCO_3^-}{\downarrow PaCO_2}\right] = \rightarrow pH$
Metabolic alkalosis	$\left[\dfrac{\uparrow HCO_3^-}{\rightarrow PaCO_2}\right] = \uparrow pH$	$\left[\dfrac{\uparrow HCO_3^-}{\uparrow PaCO_2}\right] = \rightarrow pH$

Putting It All Together

1. An excessively high level of fixed acids are present in this patient's blood. The $[HCO_3^-]$ is lower as a result of buffering fixed acids and this, in turn, lowers pH (increased $[H^+]$). Increased $[H^+]$ stimulates the respiratory system to eliminate CO_2 at a greater rate. Increased CO_2 elimination requires greater alveolar ventilation and consequentially increasing breathing frequency and tidal volumes.

2. A pH of 7.29 (acidemia) represents excessive $[H^+]$. Alveolar hyperventilation ($PaCO_2 < 35$ mm Hg) is stimulated by excessive $[H^+]$. $[H^+]$ increased because $[HCO_3^-]$ is below normal and is not adequate for buffering H^+ production. A left shift in the hydration reaction has occurred, decreasing $[H^+]$ and increasing pH. In this instance, the reason for the abnormally low HCO_3^- is not known.

3. In the information given, there is no reason given for the abnormally low $PaCO_2$. Abnormally *high* $[H^+]$ is a stimulus for hyperventilation; hyperventilation is present here ($PaCO_2 < 35$ mm Hg). But a pH of 7.52 represents abnormally *low* $[H^+]$, so a $[H^+]$ stimulus for hyperventilation does not exist. Hyperventilation in this case is the result of factors other than $[H^+]$ (e.g., excessive mechanical ventilation, central nervous system abnormality, poor pain control, anxiety, or, very commonly, hypoxemia).

4. Metabolic acidosis must ultimately be corrected by addressing its primary cause (eliminating fixed acid accumulation or replenishing HCO_3^-). In the short term, however, hyperventilation compensates for the acidosis by lowering the $PaCO_2$ below normal. If hyperventilation is required for a prolonged period of time, ventilatory muscle fatigue may occur. If blood $PaCO_2$ begins to rise in this instance (even though it may still be below normal), alveolar ventilation is decreasing, indicating that the demand for buffering by the respiratory system is greater than ventilatory reserve. At this point, ventilatory support is indicated to maintain alveolar ventilation and acid-base balance.

5. The normal ratio of $[HCO_3^-]$ to dissolved CO_2 ($PaCO_2 \times 0.03$) is 20 : 1. Ratios higher than this indicate alkalosis (increased $[HCO_3^-]$ or decreased $PaCO_2$); lower ratios indicate acidosis (decreased $[HCO_3^-]$ or increased $PaCO_2$). This is true because the remaining functions in the Henderson-Hasselbalch equation are constant.

6. $[HCO_3^-]$ = antilog(pH − 6.1) × ($PCO_2 \times 0.03$)
   $[HCO_3^-]$ = antilog(7.4 − 6.1) × (55 × 0.03)
   $[HCO_3^-]$ = antilog(1.3) × (1.65)
   $[HCO_3^-]$ = 19.95 × 1.65
   $[HCO_3^-]$ = 33.3 mEq/L

7. Since $[HCO_3^-]$ is controlled by the kidneys and does not change quickly, a rapid decrease in $PaCO_2$ to 40 mm Hg would create a state of alkalosis (above normal pH):
   pH = 6.1 + log[33.3 / (40 × 0.03)]
   pH = 6.1 + log[33.3 / 1.2)]
   pH = 6.1 + log[27.75]
   pH = 6.1 + 1.44
   pH = 7.54 (normal pH = 7.35 − 7.45)

Cases to Consider

1. This patient can be hyperventilated, which will decrease her $PaCO_2$ and reduce her $[H^+]$. An increase in pH (decreased [H+]) is directly related to a decrease in $PaCO_2$ as long as $[HCO_3^-]$ remains constant. The $PaCO_2$ required for a pH of 7.52 may be calculated with the Henderson-Hasselbalch equation:

$PaCO_2 = [HCO_3^-] / (antilog[pH - 6.1] \times 0.03)$

$PaCO_2 = 22 / (antilog[7.50 - 6.1] \times 0.03)$

$PaCO_2 = 22 / (antilog[1.4] \times 0.03)$

$PaCO_2 = 22 / (25.1 \times 0.03)$

$PaCO_2 = 29.2$ or 29 mm Hg

Attaining an arterial $PaCO_2$ of 29 mm Hg will yield a pH of 7.50 in the presence of 22 mEq/L of HCO_3^-.

2. $PaCO_2$ decreases as minute ventilation increases. (They are inversely proportional—see Chapter 8). Therefore:

$\dot{V}_{E\ initial} \times PaCO_{2\ initial} = \dot{V}_{E\ new} \times PaCO_{2\ new}$

Inserting known values for the variables,

$6.0 \times 42 = \dot{V}_{E\ new} \times 29$

$252 = \dot{V}_{E\ new} \times 29$

$\dot{V}_{E\ new} = 8.69$ L/min

If breathing frequency remains at 10 breaths/min, then tidal volume must be increased to 869 ml to achieve a $PaCO_2$ of 29 mm Hg (8,690 ml / 10 = 869 ml).

3. A simple calculation of the blood gas report's $[HCO_3^-]$ to dissolved CO_2 ratio shows:

$22 / (50 \times 0.03) = 14.67$ or about 15 : 1

The $[HCO_3^-]$ to dissolved CO_2 ratio must be 20:1 to produce a normal pH (7.40). A blood gas transcription error has probably occurred, reporting a disproportionately low $[HCO_3^-]$. Taking the patient's medical history and current clinical status into account, it is most likely that the $[HCO_3^-]$ value is erroneous.

4. $[HCO_3^-] = antilog(pH - 6.1) \times (PaCO_2 \times 0.03)$

$[HCO_3^-] = antilog(7.4 - 6.1) \times (50 \times 0.03)$

$[HCO_3^-] = antilog(1.3) \times 1.5$

$[HCO_3^-] = 19.95 \times 1.5$

$[HCO_3^-] = 29.9$ mEq/L

Chapter 11: Control of Ventilation

The Basics

1. A. Pons
   B. Medulla oblongata
   C. Spinal cord
   D. Pneumotaxic center
   E. Apneustic center
   F. Dorsal respiratory groups
   G. Ventral respiratory groups
   H. Nucleus retro-ambigualis
   I. Nucleus ambiguus
2. Progressive contraction of inspiratory muscles: 2
   Inspiratory neuronal activity completely absent; passive lung recoil occurs: 6
   Inspiratory neurons fire briefly, maintaining inspiratory muscle tone: 5
   Firing rate gradually increases from dorsal and ventral inspiratory neurons at the end of the expiratory phase: 1
   Gradual lung expansion: 3
   Inhibitory neurons turn off inspiratory signal: 4
3. Apneustic center: D
   Dorsal respiratory group: E
   Nucleus ambiguus: A
   Ventral respiratory group: C
   Pneumotaxic center: F
   Nucleus retro-ambigualis: B, E
4. B
5. C
6. C
7. Rapidly adapting irritant receptors: C
   Vagovagal reflexes: G
   Juxtacapillary receptors: A
   Peripheral proprioceptors: F
   Deflation reflex: E
   Hering-Breuer reflex: D
   Slowly adapting receptors: B
8. A
9. Main extrafusal and intrafusal fibers contract in parallel: 1
   Stretch-sensitive spindle is unloaded and its impulses cease: 5
   Main extrafusal muscle contracts, shortening nearby intrafusal muscle fibers: 4
   Spinal cord sends impulses back to the main extrafusal muscle: 3
   The spindle sensing element stretches and sends impulses over afferent nerves to the spinal cord: 2

10. C
11. D
12. B
13. A
14. [H$^+$], PCO$_2$
15. A
16. A
17. D
18. Plasma [HCO$_3^-$] increases: 5
    P$_A$CO$_2$ is chronically high: 1
    Arterial PCO$_2$ and [H$^+$] is high: 2
    Hypercapnic ventilatory drive is removed: 9
    CSF pH returns to normal: 8
    HCO$_3^-$ is retained by the kidneys: 4
    Hypoxemia is the primary ventilatory drive: 10
    CSF PCO$_2$ is high: 3
    Arterial pH returns to normal: 6
    CSF [HCO$_3^-$] increases: 7
19. D
20. B
21. A
22. C

Putting It All Together

1. Patients receiving strong analgesic medications experience central respiratory center depression that results in alveolar hypoventilation, increasing arterial carbon dioxide tension. The depressed respiratory center cannot respond to the rising PaCO$_2$, even though CSF pH is low. Hypercapnic patients with COPD also experience central respiratory center depression when high F$_I$O$_2$s remove the hypoxic breathing stimulus, allowing CSF PCO$_2$ and [H$^+$] levels to rise to excessively high levels. The two situations differ in their primary causes: analgesics directly depress ventilation, which then results in a rising PaCO$_2$. In the COPD case, the PaCO$_2$ is high to begin with, but the brain, sensing a normal pH, is not stimulated. Administering oxygen removes the hypoxic stimulus and increases $\dot{V}/\dot{Q}$ mismatch, causing further hypoventilation and CO$_2$ retention.

2. Arterial blood gases do not change from resting values during submaximal exercise. Both CO$_2$ production and O$_2$ consumption may increase dramatically during exercise, tending to increase PCO$_2$ and decrease PO$_2$. Cardiac output and ventilation also increase, appropriately matching increased needs for CO$_2$ elimination and O$_2$ delivery. Therefore blood pH remains in the normal range, and exercising tissues remain well oxygenated.

3. Abnormally high chemicals are: blood HCO$_3^-$ and CO$_2$; CSF HCO$_3^-$ and CO$_2$. Blood and CSF pH are in the normal range.

4. The increased ICP is caused by bruised, swelling brain tissue. This swelling would be aggravated by hypoventilation because high PaCO$_2$ dilates cerebral vessels, increasing blood flow to the brain. Swelling tissues may restrict venous blood flow leaving the brain, further increasing ICP. ICP may exceed arterial blood pressure, restricting blood flow and causing cerebral oxygenation to become inadequate, resulting in hypoxic brain damage. Mechanical hyperventilation reduces arterial PCO$_2$ and [H$^+$], resulting in cerebral vasoconstriction, reduced blood flow and ICP. This helps maintain appropriate arterial blood flow and oxygenation.

5. Renal retention of HCO$_3^-$ causes gradual diffusion of arterial HCO$_3^-$ ions across the blood-brain barrier to the CSF, which returns CSF [H$^+$] to normal in chronic hypercapnia. ICP may be decreased in head injury patients by mechanically hyperventilating them to reduce CSF [H$^+$]. The kidneys respond to the resulting alkalosis (from hyperventilation) by eliminating HCO$_3^-$, increasing arterial [H$^+$], and indirectly increasing ICP by increasing cerebral blood flow. In both situations, renal HCO$_3^-$ regulation eventually returns acid-base balance to normal.

Cases to Consider

1. The patient may or may not be using excessive pain medication, but the arterial blood gas report reflects normal baseline values. Although there is a slight upward trend in PO$_2$, PCO$_2$, and [H$^+$], the values represent a ventilatory status almost identical to the preoperative state. PO$_2$ and SaO$_2$ values indicate that the hypoxic drive is probably active. A normally functioning central nervous system is confirmed by the patient's alert mental status, normal breathing frequency, and normal arterial pH.

2. A decrease in mental awareness and breathing frequency indicate that the patient's PCO$_2$ (and CSF [H$^+$]) has probably risen substantially above his baseline. Oxygen is flowing at twice the rate normally required by the patient and is suppressing ventilation. The chronically hypercapnic patient is no longer being driven to breathe by hypoxia, since the SpO$_2$ is now 95% (it is at least 92% [PaO$_2$ is greater than 60 mm Hg] with the oximeter's margin of error). Reducing the oxygen flow rate to the patient's normal requirements will allow PO$_2$ to decrease below 60 mm Hg, stimulating the carotid bodies to drive ventilation. PCO$_2$ will decrease to the patient's "normal" level when alveolar ventilation increases. As CSF PCO$_2$ decreases because of diffusion along the CSF-arterial gradient, CSF [H$^+$] will decrease and remove the cause of central nervous system depression.

Chapter 12: Ventilation-Perfusion Relationships and Arterial Blood Gases

The Basics
1. D
2. A
3. A. 40 mm Hg
   B. 45 mm Hg
   C. 100 mm Hg
   D. 40 mm Hg
   E. 150 mm Hg
   F. 0 mm Hg
4. Absolute shunt: D
   Absolute deadspace: C
   Relative shunt: A
   Relative deadspace: B
   Hyperventilation: B
   Hypoventilation: A
   Low cardiac output: B
5. A
6. B
7. A
8. See the figure below.
9. See the figure below.
10. See the figure below.

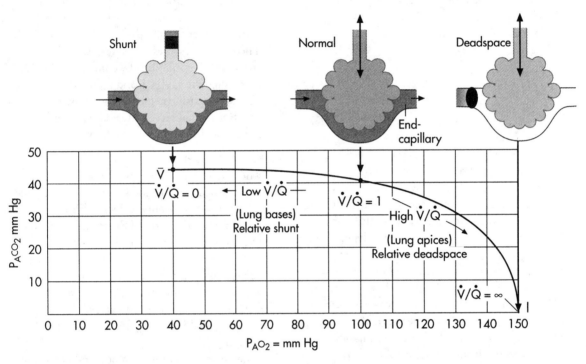

11. D
12. B
13. Hypoventilation is the reason for below normal capillary PO_2 in this figure. Alveolar hypoventilation has increased PCO_2, producing a reciprocal decrease in alveolar PO_2. Capillary PO_2 is in equilibrium with alveolar PO_2 and is decreased to the same value.
14. Atelectasis: P
    Pulmonary edema: P
    Pneumonia: P
    Ventricular septal defect: A
    Bronchial occlusion: P
    Adult respiratory distress syndrome: P
    Airway mucus plug: P
    Pneumothorax: P
    Bronchial venous admixture: A
15. B
16. C
17. D
18. A
19. If blood flow conditions remain constant, then in order to return arterial gases to their normal values (PCO_2 from 80 to 40 mm Hg and PO_2 from 50 to 100 mm Hg), minute ventilation must change to 8 L/min. This will double the CO_2 elimination (decreasing PCO_2 by half) and P_AO_2 of the normal lung.
20. $V_D/V_T = (PaCO_2 - P_ECO_2) / PaCO_2$
    $V_D/V_T = (40 - 30) / 25$
    $V_D/V_T = 10 / 25$
    $V_D/V_T = 0.40$ or 40%
    A V_D/V_T value of 40% is at the high end of the normal V_D/V_T range which is 25% to 40%.
21. C

22. $P_AO_2 = F_IO_2(PB - 47) - PaCO_2 \times 1.2$
    $P_AO_2 = 0.40(760 - 47) - 42 \times 1.2$
    $P_AO_2 = 0.40(713) - 50.4$
    $P_AO_2 = 285.2 - 50.4$
    $P_AO_2 = 234.8$

    $P(A\text{-}a)O_2 = 234.8 - 67$
    $P(A\text{-}a)O_2 = 167.8$ or 168 mm Hg

    Significant shunt is present (in normal shunt, even breathing 100% oxygen, $P(A\text{-}a)O_2$ is only 30 to 56 mm Hg).

23. D

24. Current $P_AO_2 = 0.25(760 - 47) - 35 \times 1.2$
    Current $P_AO_2 = 136.25$ mm Hg

    Needed P_AO_2 = desired PaO_2 / (PaO_2/P_AO_2)
    Needed $P_AO_2 = 70 / (50/136.25)$
    Needed $P_AO_2 = 190.75$ mm Hg

    F_IO_2 Required = $\dfrac{\text{Desired } PaO_2 / (PaO_2/P_AO_2) + PaCO_2 \times 1.2}{PB - 47}$

    F_IO_2 Required = $(190.75 + [35 \times 1.2]) / (760 - 47)$
    F_IO_2 Required = $232.75 / 713$
    F_IO_2 Required = 0.326 or 33%

25. $P_AO_2 = P_IO_2 - PaO_2$
    $P_AO_2 = 0.21(760 - 47) - 38$
    $P_AO_2 = 149.73$

    $CcO_2 = (Hb \times 1.34 \times ScO_2) + (P_AO_2 \times 0.003)$
    $CcO_2 = (14 \times 1.34 \times 1.00) + (149.73 \times 0.003)$
    $CcO_2 = 18.76 + 0.449$
    $CcO_2 = 19.21$ ml/dl

    $CaO_2 = (14 \times 1.34 \times 0.91) + (65 \times 0.003)$
    $CaO_2 = 17.07 + 0.195$
    $CaO_2 = 17.27$ ml/dl

    $C\bar{v}O_2 = (14 \times 1.34 \times 0.58) + (58 \times 0.003)$
    $C\bar{v}O_2 = 10.88 + 0.174$
    $C\bar{v}O_2 = 11.05$ ml/dl

    $\dot{Q}_S/\dot{Q}_T = (CcO_2 - CaO_2) / (CcO_2 - C\bar{v}O_2)$
    $\dot{Q}_S/\dot{Q}_T = (19.21 - 17.27) / (19.21 - 11.05)$
    $\dot{Q}_S/\dot{Q}_T = 1.94 / 8.16$
    $\dot{Q}_S/\dot{Q}_T = 0.238$ or 24%

    Twenty four percent is well above normal physiological shunt, which is about 5%.

Putting It All Together

1. Ventilation doubled while blood flow (already greater than normal) remained the same in the normal lung, increasing the $\dot{V}_A/\dot{Q}_C$ ratio back to normal. However, the overall $\dot{V}_A/\dot{Q}_C$ for both lungs is above normal because the abnormal lung receives no blood flow, but doubles its ventilation. A high $\dot{V}_A/\dot{Q}_C$ ratio indicates the presence of deadspace (ventilated, unperfused alveoli). In this situation, the high $\dot{V}_A/\dot{Q}_C$ is present in the abnormal lung and is known as absolute deadspace.

2. A. The unperfused lung represents absolute deadspace.

   B. $\dot{V}_A/\dot{Q}_C$ of the unperfused lung equals infinity ($\dot{V}_A = 8; \dot{Q}_C = 0$).

   C. Because the unperfused lung contributes no end-capillary blood flow to arterial blood flow, it also does not directly contribute to arterial gas tensions.

   D. The unperfused lung reduces breathing efficiency because half of ventilatory effort is used to ventilate alveolar space that does not communicate with blood flow. Ventilation must therefore increase (as it actually does when arterial PO_2 or PCO_2 are abnormal) just to maintain normal blood gases.

3. In order to maintain normal arterial blood oxygen concentration with relative deadspace, ventilation must increase in normal alveolar units (and, consequently, abnormal units); decreased breathing efficiency results. Impaired diaphragm movement limits the ability to sustain this increased ventilation; underventilation and hypoxemia may result.
4. The first $\dot{V}_A/\dot{Q}_C$ change occurs because alveolar ventilation is decreased in relation to perfusion. End-capillary blood leaving non-ventilated alveoli are unoxygenated, producing relative shunt (the $\dot{V}_A/\dot{Q}_C$ ratio moves toward zero). The second $\dot{V}_A/\dot{Q}_C$ change is compensatory and occurs because pulmonary vasoconstriction reduces blood flow to non-ventilated alveoli, rerouting blood flow to ventilated alveoli (the $\dot{V}_A/\dot{Q}_C$ ratio moves back toward 1.0).
5. PEEP is initiated to correct shunt-like conditions (i.e., low $\dot{V}_A/\dot{Q}_C$ ratios) to open perfused, non-ventilated alveoli. Excessively high PEEP increases the $\dot{V}_A/\dot{Q}_C$ ratio (deadspace effect) by compressing capillaries and decreasing alveolar capillary blood flow.

Cases to Consider
1. This patient has regional differences in lung compliance indicated by her spirometry results (restrictive pattern) and breath sounds (bibasilar inspiratory crackles). Ventilation-perfusion mismatch exists because of regional hypoventilation (relative shunt). Since lung compression secondary to skeletal deformity is the primary reason for her $\dot{V}_A/\dot{Q}_C$ mismatch, increasing bronchodilator therapy will not eliminate supplemental oxygen requirements in this patient.
2. The patient's right mainstem bronchus has been intubated with the endotracheal tube, effectively sealing off all ventilation to the left lung. The $\dot{V}_A/\dot{Q}_C$ condition in the left lung is absolute shunt ($\dot{V}_A/\dot{Q}_C = 0$). Calculated P(A-a)O$_2$ is:
$$P_AO_2 = F_IO_2(P_B - 47) - PaCO_2$$
$$P_AO_2 = 1.0(760 - 47) - 41$$
$$P_AO_2 = 713 - 41$$
$$P_AO_2 = 672 \text{ mm Hg}$$

$$P(A\text{-}a)O_2 = 672 - 48$$
$$P(A\text{-}a)O_2 = 624 \text{ mm Hg}$$

Chapter 13: Clinical Assessment of Acid-Base and Oxygenation Status

The Basics
1. B
2. A
3. The four steps to systematic acid-base classification are:
   Step one: Inspect the pH: Is acidemia or alkalemia present? Or is the pH normal (which side of the normal range)?
   Step two: Inspect the PaCO$_2$ (respiratory component): Can it explain the pH?
   Step three: Inspect the HCO$_3^-$ (metabolic component): Can it explain the pH?
   Step four: Check for compensation: Did the non-causative component respond appropriately?
4.

Component	Classification	Ranges
pH (arterial)	Normal	7.35–7.45
	Acidemia	< 7.35
	Alkalemia	> 7.45
PaCO$_2$ (mm Hg)	Normal ventilatory status	35–45
	Respiratory acidosis (hypoventilation)	> 45
	Respiratory alkalosis (hyperventilation)	< 35
HCO$_3^-$ (mEq/L)	Normal metabolic status	22–26
	Metabolic acidosis	< 22
	Metabolic alkalosis	> 26

5. A. Alkalemia
   B. HCO_3^-
   C. $PaCO_2$
   D. Uncompensated metabolic alkalosis
6. A. normal pH
   B. Acidic
   C. Compensated
   D. HCO_3^-
   E. Compensated respiratory acidosis
7. A. Acidemia
   B. HCO_3^-
   C. $PaCO_2$
   D. Partially compensated
8. A. Alkalemia
   B. $PaCO_2$
   C. HCO_3^-
   D. Partially compensated
9. D
10. C
11. A
12. C
13.

	pH	$PaCO_2$	$[HCO_3^-]$
Respiratory			
Acidosis (acute)	Low	High	WNL
Acidosis (chronic)	WNL	High	High
Alkalosis (acute)	High	Low	WNL
Alkalosis (chronic)	WNL	Low	Low
Metabolic			
Acidosis (acute)	Low	WNL	Low
Acidosis (chronic)	WNL	Low	Low
Alkalosis (acute)	High	WNL	High
Alkalosis (chronic)	WNL	High	High
Combined			
Acidosis	Low	High	Low
Alkalosis	High	Low	High

14. C
15. D
16. B
17. $[Cl^-]$, $[HCO_3^-]$, $[NA^+]$
18. A
19. C
20. Central chemoreceptors are stimulated: 5
    Plasma $[HCO_3^-]$ is decreased: 2
    CSF HCO_3^- diffuses into the blood: 3
    pH is normalized: 8
    Buffering of increased plasma $[H^+]$ begins: 1
    CSF pH decreases: 4
    Plasma PCO_2 and $[H_2CO_3]$ is decreased: 7
    Ventilation increases: 6
21. C
22. B

23. C
24. D
25. A
26. B
27. C
28. C
29. C
30. C
31. A
32. Decreases
33. A
34. B
35. B
36. D
37. A
38. B

Putting It All Together

1. Compensated respiratory acidosis is present. pH is on the acid of normal (but is within normal limits); PaCO$_2$ is abnormally high (the causative component tending toward acidemia); and [HCO$_3^-$] is abnormally high (the compensating component).

2. An evaluation of the present arterial blood gas values alone may lead to an interpretation of compensated metabolic alkalosis (with a pH on the alkalotic side of normal and PCO$_2$ compensating for high [HCO$_3^-$]). When the new arterial blood gas values are evaluated in the light of the patient's "normal" baseline values, it becomes apparent that alveolar hyperventilation exists. A normal PCO$_2$ level of 55 mm Hg has been decreased to 48 mm Hg. This fact, in the presence of chronically high [HCO$_3^-$], is causing the pH to move to the alkalotic side of normal. If the pH continues to increase to greater than 7.45 and if the HCO$_3^-$ remains high, uncompensated respiratory alkalosis will exist.

3. Hypoxemia stimulates peripheral chemoreceptors to increase ventilation above normal (hyperventilation). Hyperventilation is consistent with below normal PaCO$_2$ (hypocapnia) and above normal pH (alkalosis). The renal response to respiratory alkalosis is excretion of HCO$_3^-$, lowering [HCO$_3^-$] and decreasing pH to its normal range. This condition is called compensated respiratory alkalosis. Correcting prolonged hypoxemia will remove it as a stimulus for hyperventilation and PaCO$_2$ will increase. Since [HCO$_3^-$] is now below normal (and does not change quickly) metabolic acidemia will develop. Hyperventilation will thus persist because increased plasma [H$^+$] stimulates peripheral chemoreceptors, which continue to stimulate ventilation (compensating for metabolic acidosis).

4. $CaO_2 = (Hb \times 1.34 \times SaO_2) + (PaO_2 \times 0.003)$
   $CaO_2 = (17 \times 1.34 \times 0.88) + (57 \times 0.003)$
   $CaO_2 = 20.04 + 0.171$
   $CaO_2 = 20.21$ g/dl

   The arterial oxygen content is normal even with low SaO$_2$ and PaO$_2$ values. This is possible because the hemoglobin concentration is above normal and more than offsets the low SaO$_2$ and PaO$_2$ in the CaO$_2$ equation (hemoglobin is increased 13%; SaO$_2$ is decreased 11%; the effect of PaO$_2$ on CaO$_2$ is very small). Chronic hypoxemia in this patient has caused increased red blood cell production, increasing the blood hemoglobin concentration.

5. $O_2DEL = \dot{Q}_T \times (CaO_2 \times 10)$
   $CaO_2 = (Hb \times 1.34 \times SaO_2) + (PaO_2 \times 0.003)$
   $O_2ER = C(a - \bar{v})O_2 / CaO_2$
   $CaO_2 = (12 \times 1.34 \times 0.88) + (57 \times 0.003)$
   $CaO_2 = 14.15 + 0.171$
   $CaO_2 = 14.32$ g/dl

   $O_2DEL = 4.8 \times (14.32 \times 10)$
   $O_2DEL = 687.36$ or 687 ml/min

   $O_2ER = 250 / 687$
   $O_2ER = 0.364$ or 36%

   Since the patient has normal oxygen consumption, the elevated oxygen extraction (36%) ratio is the result of decreased oxygen delivery. Decreased oxygen content (14.32 g/dl) is the primary reason oxygen delivery is decreased, since cardiac output (4.8 L/min) is almost normal. SaO$_2$ and PaO$_2$ indicate that the arterial oxygen concentration is below normal (88% and 57 mm Hg, respectively). In the CaO$_2$ equation, changes in SaO$_2$ and [Hb] (12 g/dl) affect the CaO$_2$ significantly. Increasing SaO$_2$ will result in the most immediate improvement in oxygen delivery.

6. The underlying problem for both acid-base and oxygenation disturbances in these situations is stagnant hypoxia. When cardiac arrest occurs, blood circulation is at a standstill and anaerobic tissue metabolism begins in the absence of oxygen. Anaerobic metabolism produces lactic acid, which is buffered by available HCO$_3^-$. In the absence of adequate ventilation and perfusion and adequate HCO$_3^-$, PCO$_2$ rises above normal and pH decreases below normal. Aggressive chest compressions and manual ventilation restore PO$_2$

to normal or higher values while PCO_2 drops below normal. Below normal PCO_2 is useful in this situation to counteract extremely low pH. $[HCO_3^-]$ is so low that hyperventilation may still have limited effect in normalizing the pH.

Cases To Consider
1. Ventilation is adequate for this patient. Although decreased from 80 mm Hg, the $PaCO_2$ remains high with a normal pH because the $[HCO_3^-]$ is (chronically) above normal. This means that this person's normal stable arterial blood gases have probably been achieved. Increasing alveolar ventilation further could result in alkalosis.
2. The arterial blood gas results show a combined respiratory and metabolic acidosis (pH < 7.35). The respiratory component, PCO_2 at 47 mm Hg, is on the acidic side of its normal range of 35 to 45 mm Hg. The metabolic component, $[HCO_3^-]$ (20 mEq/L), is also contributing to acidosis since it is below its normal range of 22 to 26 mEq/L. The cause of the acid-base disturbance is alveolar hypoventilation and excessive loss of HCO_3^- from diarrhea. The primary cause of hypoxemia is relative shunt, or $\dot{V}_A/\dot{Q}_C$ mismatch. Therapy must be directed at improving hypoxemia with supplemental oxygen and improving the low $\dot{V}_A/\dot{Q}_C$ ratio by relieving airway obstruction with inhaled bronchodilators. These strategies will not only increase PaO_2 but will allow the patient to increase alveolar ventilation, decreasing $PaCO_2$ and improving pH. $[HCO_3^-]$ will improve when the diarrhea is controlled.

Chapter 14: Functional Anatomy of the Cardiovascular System

The Basics
1. Pericardial fluid: 5
   Parietal pericardium: 6
   Ventricle: 1
   Myocardium: 3
   Epicardium: 4
   Fibrous pericardium: 7
   Endocardium: 2
2. C
3. Anterior
4. Left ventricle: 10
   Right ventricle: 4
   Left atrium: 8
   Right atrium: 2
   Pulmonic valve: 5
   Tricuspid valve: 3
   Aortic valve: 11
   Bicuspid valve: 9
   Vena cavae: 1
   Pulmonary artery: 6
   Aorta: 12
   Lungs: 7
5. B
6. Trabeculae carneae: C
   Chordae tendineae: F
   Myocardium: B
   Foramen ovale: G
   Papillary muscles: E
   Fibrous annuli: H
   Pericardial fluid: D
   Visceral pericardium: A
7. B
8. Diastole
9. A
10. C
11. D
12. A. Sinoatrial node
    B. Atrioventricular node
    C. Atrioventricular bundle
    D. Left and right bundle branches
    E. Purkinje fibers
    F. Apex
    G. Interventricular septum
    H. Left ventricle
    I. Left atrium
13. A
14. A
15. B
16. C
17. Muscle fiber: D
    Sarcolemma: I
    T-tubule: H
    Sarcoplasmic reticulum: F
    Myofibril: G
    Myosin: C
    Actin: B
    Sarcomere: A
    Z-line: E
18. Acetylcholine stimulates the sarcolemma: 1
    Tropomyosin strands slide into actin grooves: 3
    Myosin cross-bridges pull the actin filament toward the sarcomere's center: 5
    ATP molecules bind with the myosin cross-bridge and pull it to its resting position: 6
    Sarcoplasmic reticulum releases Ca^{++} ions: 2
    Energized myosin cross-bridges bind with actin sites: 4
19. D

20. C
21. A
22. B
23. Left ventricle: D
    Conducting arteries: G
    Arterioles: A
    Microcirculation: C
    Anastomosis: F
    Veins: B
    Pulse pressure: E
24. B
25. A
26. C
27. C
28. Increases
29. Increase
30. A
31. A
32. D
33. B

Putting It All Together

1. B
2. Ventricular pressures rise enough to open semilunar valves: 3
   The ventricles contract against closed semilunar valves: 2
   Ventricular pressures build, forcefully closing the atrioventricular valves: 1
   Atrial pressures fall as blood drains into the ventricles: 8
   Back flow of blood into ventricles is stopped abruptly, causing dilation and recoil of the aorta and pulmonary artery: 6
   The ventricles relax; their pressures fall; and semilunar valves snap shut: 5
   Ventricular contraction closes the atrioventricular valves: 10
   The ejection period occurs: 4
   The atria contracts, slightly distending ventricular walls: 9
   Ventricular pressures fall and atrioventricular valves open: 7
3. Dicrotic notch (in aortic and pulmonary artery waveforms): 6
   First heart sound: 10
   Second heart sound: 5
   Isovolumetric contraction: 2
   Isovolumetric relaxation: 7
   Atrial kick: 9
4. Sympathetic peripheral vasoconstriction redirects blood flow to larger central vessels in acute blood loss. Redirected blood meets less resistance in larger vessels that lead to central organs, increasing their blood flow.
5. Right ventricular failure is the result of ineffective ventricular pumping. This condition causes a "back up" of venous blood flow and increases RAP. Increased RAP results in increased pressure throughout the systemic venous system. Exposed to abnormally high pressures, capillary beds leak fluid into interstitial spaces and cause tissue swelling (edema).
6. C
7. Tracheal suctioning, selection "C," is the only situation that does not mimic or cause sympathetic stimulation, thereby increasing the heart rate. Tracheal suctioning results in bradycardia (slow heart rate) because it easily stimulates the parasympathetic nerves lining the trachea. Parasympathetic stimulation is a cause of bradycardia.
8. Jugular venous distension, pedal edema, and abdominal ascites are the result of right ventricular failure. When right ventricular pumping action is inadequate, peripheral fluid accumulation occurs. Diuresis decreases overall blood volume through renal fluid elimination; venous blood flow then decreases, more closely matching right ventricular pumping ability. As blood volume becomes more appropriate for right ventricular pumping ability, venous fluid accumulation subsides.
9. If adequate perfusion is necessary for a normal urine production rate, then decreasing perfusion decreases urine production. Left ventricular failure is characterized by low systemic perfusion and would therefore cause low urine output.

Cases to Consider

1. A needle inserted into the pleural space of this patient's right thorax will relieve a tension pneumothorax. The absence of breath sounds over the upper right lung area and a left-shifted PMI point to a collapsed right upper lobe and increased pressure in the right hemithorax. The thin-walled bullae in this patient's lungs have predisposed them to spontaneous rupture and subsequent lung collapse. Pressurization of the right hemithorax occurred as inspired air was trapped between the affected lobe and the parietal pleura. The needle decompresses the lung, momentarily improving cardiovascular symptoms. Subsequent placement of a chest tube will allow re-expansion of the affected lobe and improve the hypoxemia that resulted from blood being shunted through the collapsed lobe. As hypoxemia improves, respiratory distress and tachycardia, both signs of hypoxemia, will improve. Decreasing pressure in the thorax will also increase venous return, raise cardiac output, and normalize blood pressure.

2. This patient exhibits signs of congestive right heart failure. Pedal edema and JVD indicate that right heart pumping is failing to keep pace with the return flow of systemic venous blood. The abnormally high CVP (normal is about 0 mm Hg) also indicates a "backup" of blood returning to the right atrium. Starting this patient on a diuretic will reduce the blood volume to a quantity manageable for right heart pumping ability. As the diuretic eliminates fluid volume, the patient's weight will also return to baseline.

Chapter 15: Cardiac Electrophysiology

The Basics
1. Positive, negative
2. B
3. D
4. B
5. K^+, Ca^{++}, Na^+
6. Out of, into
7. A
8. A
9. D
10.

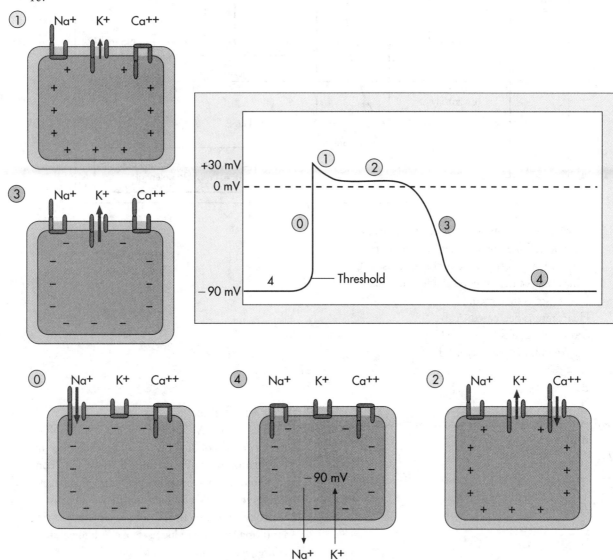

11. Depolarization: B
    Repolarization: E
    Action potential: F
    Threshold potential: C
    Refractory: A
    Excitability: G
    Hyperpolarized: D
12. B
13. C
14. D
15.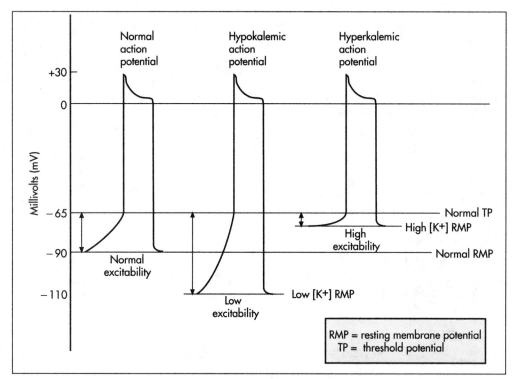
16. Cardiac cell membrane is more excitable: A
    Cardiac cell membrane is less excitable: B
    Amplitude of action potential is increased: B
    Amplitude of action potential is reduced: A
    Heart rate is increased: C
    Heart rate is decreased: A, B
    Stroke volume is increased: C
    Stroke volume is decreased: B
17. B
18. B
19. A
20. Automaticity, rhythmicity, excitability, contractility
21. C
22. C
23. C
24. A
25. A
26. B
27. B
28. D

Putting It All Together

1. Normally, the AV conduction rate is slower than the SA node conduction rate. This difference in conduction rates allows time for the atria to contract and fill the ventricles before they contract. An increased AV conduction rate would cause ventricular contraction before complete ventricular filling, causing reduced stroke volume and, consequently, low cardiac output.

2. Stimulation of cardiac muscle beta receptor sites increases heart rate and contractility. These changes would normally be reflected in the patient's pulse rate, pulse strength, and blood pressure.
3. Heart rate will be determined by the AV node, a lower order pacemaker, since it has the highest spontaneous depolarization rate next to the SA node. The heart rate will be equal to the firing rate of the AV node, 40 to 60 beats/min, lower than the SA node rate of 70 to 80 beats/min.
4. Bachmann's bundle conducts the SA node impulse directly to the left atrium at the same rate it is conducted to the AV node. If the conduction rate in Bachmann's bundle were reduced, the left atrium would contract after right atrial contraction and would be asynchronous with the left ventricle.
5. The main effect of calcium channel blockers is to decrease cardiac muscle contractile force. Decreased myocardial contractile force results in decreased stroke volume. Blood pressure would be compromised even further in an already hypotensive patient.
6. Severe hypokalemia may result in cardiac arrest; in less severe hypokalemic states, a decreased heart rate occurs.

A Case to Consider
1. An inotropic drug will increase cardiac contractility. Increased contractility improves stroke volume and cardiac output, relieving venous congestion. It may also improve kidney perfusion, increasing urine output and reducing blood volume. Adequate calcium induction into myocardial cells during the action potential is essential for muscle contraction. Digitalis increases contractility by increasing calcium stores in cardiac fiber.

Chapter 16: The Electrocardiogram and Cardiac Arrhythmias

The Basics
1. C
2.

(From Thibodeau GA, Patton KT: *Anatomy and physiology*, ed 3, St Louis, 1996, Mosby.)

3. P wave: B, J
   QRS complex: E, G
   T wave: A, I
   P-R interval: D
   ST segment: F
   Q-T interval: C
4. A
5. C

6.

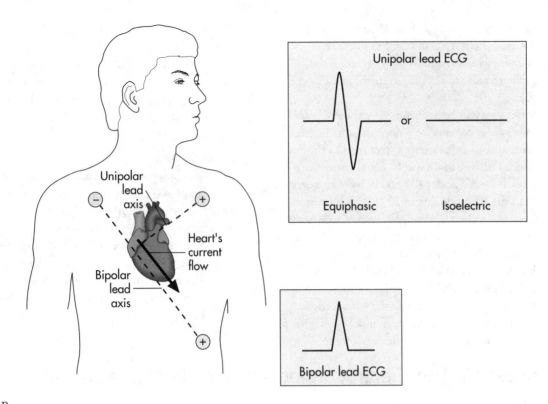

7. B
8. C
9. A
10. Right arm, left arm, right arm, left leg, left arm, left leg
11. II, I, III
12. D
13.

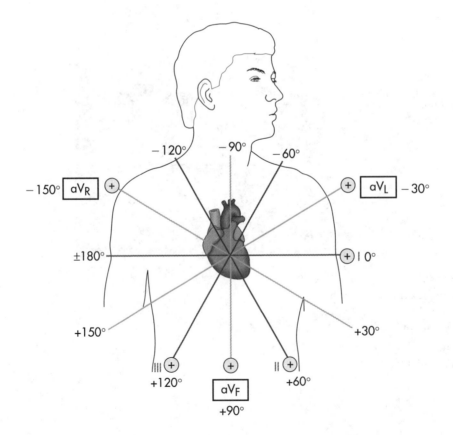

14. D

15. Steps in ECG analysis are as follows. Step one: Identify specific waves. Step two: Analyze QRS complexes (rate, rhythm, QRS shape). Step three: Analyze P waves (rate, rhythm, shape). Step four: Assess atrial-ventricular relationship (ratio of P waves to QRS complexes; location of P wave with respect to QRS complex; P-R interval).
16. B
17. C
18. More P waves than QRS complexes: B
    P wave polarity opposite of expected: F
    Wide QRS complex: C
    P wave follows QRS complex: E
    PR interval greater than 0.2 seconds: A
    Two QRSs of different polarity: D
19. C
20. B
21. C
22. A
23. Atrial flutter: C
    Atrial fibrillation: F
    Junctional escape rhythm: B
    Premature junctional contraction: A
    Junctional tachycardia: D
    Paroxysmal supraventricular tachycardia: E
24. D
25. D
26. B
27. Torsades de pointes: A
    Ventricular fibrillation: D
    Bigeminy: F
    Ventricular tachycardia: B
    Multifocal PVCs: E
    Circus re-entry: C
28. A
29. B
30. C

Putting It All Together

1. Negative QRS deflection in lead I indicates that depolarizing current is flowing to the right of a vertical axis at the heart's center. Negative QRS deflection in lead aV_F indicates depolarizing current is also flowing superior to a horizontal axis through the heart's center. Comparing QRS complexes from both leads, it is apparent that an extreme right axis deviation to the right upper quadrant exists.
2. C
3. C
4. When retrograde P waves are present, P waves appear after QRS complexes, which is opposite of normal. Retrograde P waves indicate that the depolarizing electrical impulse is reaching the ventricles before it reaches the atria, causing ventricular contraction to occur before atrial contraction. Ventricular filling is reduced under these conditions, and cardiac output will decrease.
5. On an ECG, "f" waves indicate that an atrial arrhythmia, atrial fibrillation, is present. P waves are not present in atrial fibrillation, since multiple atrial foci are firing in random order. Widened QRS complexes indicate that the impulse for ventricular contraction originates in the ventricles. Since the QRS complexes are similar in shape, there is only one ventricular ectopic focus pacing the heart. A second arrhythmia, complete heart (third degree AV) block also exists. Because all QRS complexes are widened, all impulses for ventricular depolarization originate in the ventricles; none are conducted from the atria. A heart rate of 50 beats/min is also consistent with a rhythm paced in the ventricles.
6. In this situation, a heart with normal muscle mass has a normally left-positioned ventricle now positioned on the right. Assuming normal placement of ECG leads, the ECG will reflect a right axis deviation in the +90° to +180° quadrant. This occurs because the mean cardiac vector still points in the direction of mean electrical activity, which has been affected by the (repositioned) greater muscle mass of the left heart.
7. Although ventricular filling time and cardiac output are significantly reduced, some perfusion still exists in ventricular tachycardia. In ventricular fibrillation, the random firing of multiple foci results in unorganized muscular contraction and cardiac output ceases altogether; reducing perfusion to zero.
8. A depolarizing impulse that originates near the bifurcation of the bundle of His is more likely to be conducted along normal ventricular pathways (the bundle of His and Purkinje fibers). An impulse originating lower in the ventricles will have a lengthy conduction time and trace a very abnormal pathway.
9. Both measurements use the same grid, which is based on 1 mm squares. Conduction voltage is represented on an ECG by the amplitude (*height*) of the wave (10 small squares = 1 mv). Conduction time is represented by the *length* of a wave (1 small square = 0.04 sec).

Cases to Consider

1. This patient's syncope and hypotension are related to atrial fibrillation. Hypotension in this case is probably not related to hypovolemia since the patient's weight is slightly above baseline. Rather, it is the result of low cardiac output caused by a high ventricular rate of 160 to 180 beats/min. (Eight to nine QRS complexes per 3 second interval means there are 16 to 18 in 6 seconds and 160 to 180 in 1 minute.) The absence of P waves and an irregular, "wavy" baseline indicate that atrial fibrillation is present and the atrial impulse rate is probably 300 to 600 per minute (the refractory AV node is allowing conduction of only part of the atrial impulses to the ventricles). The patient's atrial fibrillation is the product of progressive congestive heart failure that has enlarged the atria, increasing conduction time in internodal pathways. The irritability of atrial tissue has increased, and many ectopic foci have developed as a result. The excessive ventricular rate can be reduced (which will increase cardiac output and blood pressure) by administering calcium channel blockers. Giving the patient quinidine will reduce atrial irritability, resulting in a lower atrial impulse and lower conduction rate to the ventricles. Anticoagulant therapy may also be indicated to inhibit the development of atrial thromboemboli from blood pooling.

2. Wide QRS complexes indicate that depolarizing impulses originate in the ventricles. The presence of P waves indicates that the SA node is functional, but, since all QRS complexes are wide, no SA node impulses reach the ventricles. This is known as third-degree block. In this arrhythmia, the ventricles are self-pacing in a ventricular escape rhythm. Because the ventricular rhythm is an escape rhythm, there is no indication that increased ventricular irritability exists. For this reason, lidocaine therapy is inappropriate. Third degree block may be treated with parasympatholytic (parasympathetic blocking) or beta-adrenergic drugs or with an artificial pacemaker.

Chapter 17: Control of Cardiac Output and Hemodynamics

The Basics

1. B
2. C
3. A
4. C
5. D
6. D
7.

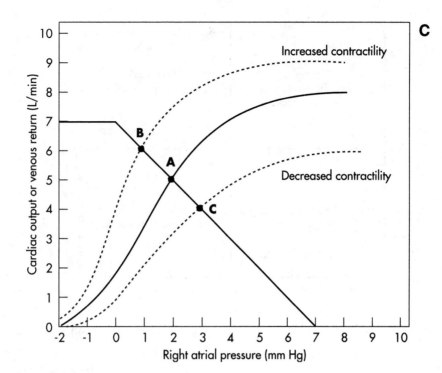

8. B
9. C
10. C
11. B
12. Central venous pressure <6 mm Hg
    Pulmonary artery pressure (systolic/diastolic): 20-30/6-15 mm Hg
    Mean pulmonary artery pressure: 10-20 mm Hg
    Pulmonary capillary wedge pressure: 4-12 mm Hg
    Cardiac output: 4-8 L/min
    Systemic arterial pressure (systolic/diastolic): 120/80 mm Hg
    Mean systemic arterial pressure: 80-100 mm Hg
13. A
14. C
15. D
16. Cardiac index (CI): CO/BSA
    Stroke volume (SV): CO/HR
    Stroke index (SI): SV/BSA
    Systemic vascular resistance (SVR): (MAP − RAP)/CO × 80
    Pulmonary vascular resistance (PVR): (MPAP − PCWP)/CO × 80
    Left ventricular stroke work index (LVSWI): SI × (MAP − PCWP) × 0.0136
    Right ventricular stroke work index (RVSWI): SI × (MPAP − CVP) × 0.0136
17. A
18. D
19. A

Answer Key 173

20.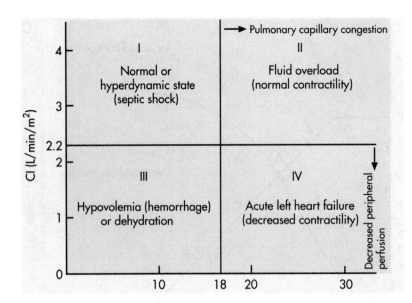

21. C
22. B
23. A

Putting It All Together

1. C
2. D
3. Systemic vasodilation results in reduced SVR. When SVR decreases, ventricular afterload (outflow resistance) also decreases. As shown on the vascular function curve, low vascular resistance results in increased cardiac output.
4. Decreasing the amount of calcium available to myocardial fiber has a negative inotropic effect on the heart. Decreased calcium results in reduced contractility. Myocardial oxygen consumption is also decreased, since it is proportional to myocardial contractility.
5. A high level of PEEP will decrease cardiac output. It does so by decreasing the pressure gradient between the aorta and the right atrium (returning venous blood encounters intrathoracic pressure that is closer to mean aortic pressure). This means that the rate of flow for blood returning to the heart is reduced as well. If venous return is reduced, so is right atrial pressure. On the cardiac function curve, a reduction in right atrial pressure (ventricular preload) causes a reduction in cardiac output.
6. Left ventricular failure results in a decreased ejection fraction and increased ventricular end-diastolic volume. If blood flow to the left atrium remains normal, left atrial and left ventricular end-diastolic pressures (measured by the PCWP) will increase. Pulmonary capillaries subjected to pressures greater than 18 mm Hg become "leaky," permitting fluid accumulation in the alveoli (pulmonary edema). In situations where the alveolar-capillary membrane is damaged (such as adult respiratory distress syndrome), its normal impermeability to fluid is lost and pulmonary edema occurs at normal PCWP.
7. It is possible for CVP, MPAP, PCWP, and MAP to all be elevated with jugular venous distension. If MAP were elevated, the increase in aortic pressure could cause upstream increases in left ventricular end-diastolic pressure (PCWP), if contractility fails to increase proportionally. This would result in increased pulmonary vascular pressure (MPAP) and right ventricular end-diastolic pressure (CVP). The cause for jugular venous distension could begin at other points: increased PCWP (e.g., left ventricular failure), increased MPAP (e.g., hypoxic pulmonary hypertension), or increased CVP (right ventricular failure).

Cases to Consider

1. Dopamine is an inotropic drug; it will improve myocardial contractility. Decreased contractility is indicated here by low cardiac output (CO) and LVSWI. Low CO secondary to pumping failure caused an increased PCWP of 16 mm Hg (normal is 4 to 12 mm Hg). The PAP and CVP may also be increased from the upstream effects of elevated PCWP. Increasing the myocardial contractility will raise the cardiac output; greater cardiac output will help assure adequate perfusion and tissue oxygenation. Inotropic agents such as dopamine must be used judiciously since, along with increasing contractility, they also increase myocardial oxygen consumption.

2. The inotropic drug produced the desired effect in decreasing PCWP and improving CO and LVSWI. Diastolic PAP pressure has trended downward along with PCWP, but systolic PAP remains above normal. Since the patient's medical history includes chronic hypoxemia, hypoxemic pulmonary vasoconstriction is causing increased right ventricular afterload. This is reflected in an elevated systolic PAP of 42 mm Hg. Providing supplemental oxygen will decrease pulmonary vascular resistance and improve tissue oxygenation.

Chapter 18: Cardiopulmonary Response to Exercise in Health, Disease, and Aging

The Basics
1. D
2. A
3. A
4. C
5. D
6. Greater than
7. B
8. Exercise begins to intensify: 1
   Oxygen consumption increases: 3
   Pulse pressure rises significantly: 5
   Contracting muscles consume increasing amounts of ATP: 2
   Cardiac output increases: 4
   Skeletal capillaries are recruited in working muscles: 6
9. C
10. A
11. B
12. D
13. C
14. A
15. Decreases
16. D
17. B
18. A
19. C
20. D

21.

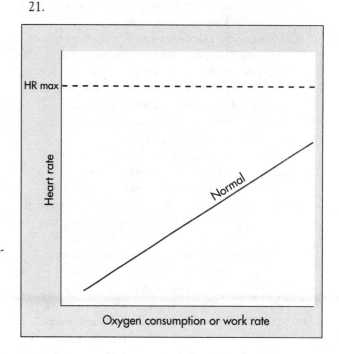

22. B
23. B
24. C
25. C
26. D
27. A
28. C

Putting It All Together

1. A chronically hypercapnic patient is unable to generate enough alveolar ventilation to maintain blood CO_2 within normal limits, even at rest. Metabolism of carbohydrates such as sugar and starch produces more CO_2 than does metabolism of fats. A predominantly carbohydrate diet may produce excessive CO_2. The additional work of breathing imposed on the patient by additional CO_2 may be intolerably high and lead to respiratory distress.

2. The time required for "repayment" of oxygen debt is dependent on an individual's capacity for hyperventilation after exercise. Ventilatory impairment will lengthen the time required to replenish oxygen stores and aerobic synthesis of ATP. Blood pH will remain low for a longer period of time because the CO_2 elimination rate (and metabolic acidosis buffering capability) is low.

3. Cardiac capacity is the factor that normally limits exercise. The primary determinant of cardiac capacity is maximum attainable heart rate.

Because the ejection fraction is decreased, stroke volume is also decreased. In an effort to maintain appropriate cardiac output (and oxygen delivery), the heart must now increase its rate to compensate for low stroke volume. In this situation, maximum exercise will be reached sooner (and at a lower level) than normal because maximum attainable heart rate has been reached prematurely. Since HRR is calculated by subtracting observed maximum heart rate from predicted maximum heart rate, this individual's HRR at maximum exercise is zero. The O_2 pulse is below normal in this situation because the heart rate will be high in relation to the oxygen consumption rate.

4. Physically fit people have greater amounts of cardiac muscle mass, greater contractility, and, therefore, higher stroke volumes than those who are less physically fit. Since cardiac output is the product of heart rate and stroke volume, an increased stroke volume requires a lower heart rate to maintain resting cardiac output.

5. In healthy individuals, cardiac output increases in response to increased oxygen consumption, and higher levels of exercise are attainable. In cardiac disease, cardiac output does not keep pace with tissue oxygen demands. Therefore the rate of oxygen consumption decreases and plateaus because oxygen delivery is inadequate to meet the increasing oxygen demand of the tissues.

6. The HRR of a patient with severe COPD is greater than normal because exercise in severe COPD is limited by minute ventilation, instead of heart rate. Because of this, maximal exercise is reached before maximal heart rate is achieved.

Cases to Consider

1. From the information given, these exercise test results must be interpreted as normal. Actual maximal heart rate is equal to predicted at 150/min (220 − 70 = 150). Respiratory exchange ratio (R = $\dot{V}CO_2/\dot{V}O_2$) increased as it should since carbon dioxide elimination ($\dot{V}CO_2$) increased at a greater rate than oxygen consumption ($\dot{V}O_2$). A breathing reserve of 30% is within normal limits (normal = 20% to 50%). HRR is calculated by subtracting the observed maximal heart rate from the predicted maximal heart rate. This patient's predicted and observed maximal heart rates are equal. Therefore HRR is zero, which is the normal value.

2. Although different limitations are present, both cardiac disease (perfusion limitation) and pulmonary disease (ventilation limitation) will cause the patient to reach anaerobic threshold at relatively low work rates. In both disease states, the V_D/V_T ratio is high, but for different reasons. The high V_D/V_T ratio with exercise in cardiac disease is the result of poor pulmonary perfusion, which means that nonperfused alveoli are ventilated (deadspace ventilation). In pulmonary disease, the high V_D/V_T ratio is caused by baseline ventilation-perfusion mismatch so that increased ventilation results in deadspace ventilation increases that are greater than increases in alveolar ventilation. Overall, this patient's exercise limitation is due to cardiac disease because test results indicate: a greater than normal ventilatory reserve, a low O_2 pulse, and a maximum heart rate reached at low work rate. Ventilatory reserve is higher than normal in cardiac disease because exercise is limited by cardiac output, and maximal exercise is reached before ventilatory reserve is exhausted. In an attempt to maintain cardiac output with low stroke volume, increases in heart rate during exercise are disproportionately high relative to increases in work rate. For this reason, maximum heart rate is reached earlier than normal. The O_2 pulse ($\dot{V}O_2$/HR) is low because the increase in heart rate during exercise is out of proportion to increases in oxygen consumption.

Chapter 19: Renal Regulation of Fluid, Electrolyte, and Acid-Base Balance

The Basics
1. A. Peritubular capillaries
   B. Vasa recta
   C. Loop of Henle
   D. Efferent arteriole
   E. Juxtaglomerular apparatus
   F. Afferent arteriole
   G. Distal convoluted tubule
   H. Renal corpuscle
   I. Proximal convoluted tubule
2. B
3. A
4. D
5. D
6. High, low
7. C

8. B
9. D
10. A
11. B
12. Increases
13. D
14. D
15. Decreases, increases
16. Bowman's capsule: 1
    Distal convoluted tubule: 4
    Proximal convoluted tubule: 2
    Collecting duct: 5
    Loop of Henle: 3
17. A
18. Decreases, decreases
19. A
20. B
21. B
22. C
23. C
24. B
25. A
26. A
27. D
28. D
29. B
30. Greater than, greater than
31. C
32. A. Hypokalemia, alkalosis
    B. Hyperkalemia, acidosis
33. B
34. C
35. A
36. C

Putting It All Together

1. Osmotic pressure changes, and water is reabsorbed from the filtrate: 7
   Sodium is actively reabsorbed from the distal tubular filtrate: 6
   Angiotensin II is formed: 4
   Extracellular fluid volume falls below normal: 1
   Adrenal glands secrete aldosterone: 5
   Extracellular fluid volume is restored toward normal: 8
   Macula densa cells of the juxtaglomerular apparatus secrete renin: 3
   Renal blood flow decreases: 2
2. Renin: Decreased
   Aldosterone: Decreased
   Atrial natriuretic hormone: Increased
   Antidiuretic hormone: Decreased
3. A patient with congestive heart failure also exhibits low blood pressure and, consequently, low perfusion. Low renal perfusion pressure stimulates the secretion of aldosterone and antidiuretic hormone. These two substances cause increased water reabsorption, which increases overall blood volume.
4. C
5. Metabolic alkalosis, as may occur with nasogastric suction and/or diuretic use, causes hypochloremia. Hypochloremia results in greater than normal secretion of potassium (and hydrogen) ions in exchange for sodium ions (secondary active secretion mechanism). Administering potassium chloride allows sodium ions to be reabsorbed with chloride ions (primary active transport). It also replenishes potassium ions depleted in the exchange for sodium ions.
6. About 65% of filtrate potassium is reabsorbed into the blood by co-transport with sodium. This means that if reabsorption of sodium is blocked, reabsorption of potassium will be blocked as well.
7. Kidneys of people with chronic acidosis (as occurs with chronic hypercapnia) produce large amounts of ammonia molecules to buffer excess hydrogen ions. Ammonia molecules combine with the hydrogen ions to produce positively charged ammonium ions. The formation of ammonium ions eliminates a large amount of free negatively charged chloride ions and hypochloremia results. Reabsorption of sodium usually requires simultaneous reabsorption of chloride. In the absence of sufficient amounts of chloride ions, hydrogen and potassium ions are secreted and hypokalemia alkalemia result.
8. The kidney preferentially reabsorbs sodium over other electrolytes. When potassium ions are not available to exchange for sodium ions, greater than normal amounts of hydrogen ions are secreted to reabsorb the sodium ions. The fall in hydrogen ion concentration results in alkalosis.
9. Potassium chloride may be necessary for a patient with severe potassium depletion in order to avoid potentially lethal cardiac arrhythmias. However, an alkalotic patient may be hypokalemic because potassium ions replace intracellular hydrogen ions. This results in low plasma potassium concentration. As the underlying cause of alkalosis is corrected, hydrogen ions replace intracellular potassium ions, which move back into the plasma.

If supplemental potassium chloride is being infused, an excessively high level of plasma potassium could result, leading to cardiac arrhythmias.

A Case to Consider

Arterial blood gas analysis is indicated by the patient's pulmonary history and current deterioration alone. This patient has a compromised ventilatory status even at baseline; ventilatory function was below baseline on admission and may have deteriorated since then. Elevated BUN and Cr may indicate renal failure. The fact that these values have risen since admission indicates worsening renal function. A repeat arterial blood gas analysis will probably reveal a combined respiratory and metabolic acidosis due to acute CO_2 retention and renal failure. The anticipated blood gas results will also indicate that this patient's significantly compromised ventilatory status is unable to tolerate the additional ventilatory work load of metabolic acidosis. Mechanical ventilation will be required to support an overburdened ventilatory pump and compensate for metabolic acidosis.